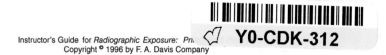
Instructor's Guide

for

RADIOGRAPHIC EXPOSURE
Principles & Practice

Jerry Ellen Wallace, MEd, RT(R)

 F. A. DAVIS COMPANY • PHILADELPHIA

Instructor's Guide for *Radiographic Exposure: Principles & Practice*
Copyright © 1996 by F.A. Davis Company

F. A. DAVIS COMPANY
1915 Arch Street
Philadelphia, PA 19103

Last digit indicates print number: 10 9 8 7 6 5 4 3 2 1

Printed in the United States of America

ISBN 0-8036-0214-6

TABLE OF CONTENTS

INTRODUCTION

This Instructor's Guide correlates with the textbook, *Radiographic Exposure: Principles & Practice*, written by Jerry Ellen Wallace and published by F.A. Davis Co., Inc. This guide has many useful features that make it easy for instructors and students to use the textbook.

The guide is written as if the textbook will be used chronologically from Chapter 1 through Chapter 18; however, there are some variations that give instructors the flexibility to use the text to correlate with the ability level of the individual class of students, the students' clinical experience, and also the other academic material the students are attempting to master at the same time. Some of the variations are presented in the section on variations.

USING THE TEXTBOOK

Each of the chapters in the text is designed to be used as an instructional unit. An instructional unit consists of several lessons in which the material in the book is reviewed and enhanced, after which the instructor gives a unit test that assesses the students' mastery of the material. This guide divides each chapter or instructional unit into the number of lessons required to present the material in a class using a 45- to 60-minute class. A suggested lesson plan for each class period is included in this guide. Each lesson plan contains:
1. The goal for the lesson.
2. The reading assignment from the text which correlates with the lesson.
3. Objectives for the lesson.
4. Suggestions on how to incorporate the activities in the text with the lesson.
5. Test questions for the lesson that can be used for the unit test; these are different questions from those that are in the textbook.

PLANNING THE COURSE

The course as suggested in this guide requires about 65 hours of class time with additional time devoted to laboratory activities. More time is required to use Appendix A, the math review, before beginning the course. More time is also necessary if time is devoted to the unit reviews in the text that can be used to reinforce difficult material or to give individual students

1

more practice if they need it. Additional time is also required if a general review is used at the end of the course.

ORDER OF PRESENTATION

The text is divided into sections beginning with an introductory section in Chapters 1 and 2 on the four radiographic qualities and the production and properties of x-rays. It is highly recommended that this section be presented first. After this first section, Sections 2 through 5 can be used in any order. Some suggestions on how to do this are presented in the following variations. Section 6 reviews and expands on the previous sections and should be used last.

VARIATIONS

Incorporating the Math Review

Begin the course using Appendix A, the math review. The time required to present this material in class depends on the ability of the class of students. Appendix A of this guide is a test to be used to assess the students' math ability. This can be used before the beginning of the course to see if a math review is required, or it can be used after a classroom math review to assess the students' mastery of math.

Chapter 1 Variations

The instructor may want to vary the amount of time spent in class on Chapter 1, which is an introduction to exposure.

Tables 1-1 and 1-2 introduce the students to some basic terminology and also to some basic equipment used in clinical education. Depending on how much experience the students have already had with this terminology and equipment, the instructor may want to devote more time to lab activities to acquaint the students with equipment used in clinical education.

Primary Exposure Factors Before Distortion

Section 2 is devoted to the radiographic quality of distortion which relates to the material the students are learning in early positioning and procedures classes. However, it may fit better into the program's master plan to have the students learn about the primary exposure factors in Section 3 before the section on distortion. There should be no problem presenting section 3 before Section 2. In this case, it would be a good idea

2

to use the material from Chapter 3, pages 25-28, which discusses introductory distance terminology before beginning Chapter 6 on the Inverse Square Law. Activity 3.A will give the student practice in using distance terms and calculating the distances.

Variations on Chapters 12 and 13

Some master plans require a separate course on radiographic film processing. Film processing is presented late in the text in Chapter 12 and part of Chapter 13 in the section devoted to recorded detail. This material can easily be broken out and used for a course on film processing. Chapter 12 begins with elements of film construction supported by review activities 12.A and 12.B. Types of film are discussed next, along with activity 12.C. Then the sections and systems of the processor are discussed along with processor chemicals. Activities 12.D and 12.E are used with this material. Chapter 12 ends with material on the characteristic curve and activity 12.F. Some instructors may want to save the material on the characteristic curve to use in a course on quality assurance. Pages 158-165 in Chapter 13 present material on the construction and function of intensifying screens. This is usually incorporated into a course on film processing; this material, along with activities 13.A and 13.B, can be used at the appropriate time in the processing course.

USING THE ACTIVITIES

The activities in the textbook consist of a variety of practice, reinforcement, review, and laboratory procedures. The activities included are drawing assignments, math practice, fill-in, multiple choice questions, laboratory activities not requiring exposure with x-ray, laboratory activities requiring exposure with x-ray, practice with using charts, word searches, and crossword puzzles.

As students read the material in the text, they are instructed to perform the activities at appropriate times. When listed in the text, these activities relate *only* to the pages the students have read since the last activity. They do not incorporate other material unless the chapter is specifically a review. This is convenient when using any of the variations listed above because as portions of the text are used in a different chronological order, the activities can be moved right along with the text.

The activities can be used for homework assignments, classroom assignments, group activities, and laboratory activities. In the lesson plans, the activities that correlate with that lesson are listed, and the type of activity is indicated.

SECTION I
IMAGE QUALITIES AND IMAGE PRODUCTION

CHAPTER 1
THE FOUR RADIOGRAPHIC QUALITIES

Chapter 1 is an introductory chapter designed to acquaint students with the four radiographic qualities of density, contrast, recorded detail, and distortion. This is an important foundation for the rest of the text. This chapter is written in an easy-to-read style and the activities are not very challenging. This is so the students will not be intimidated early in the course. This chapter is different from the other chapters in the book because Lesson 1-1 is the only lesson used for this chapter. It is suggested that the class session be informal.

LESSON 1-1: THE FOUR RADIOGRAPHIC QUALITIES

Goal

Students will begin to recognize the four radiographic qualities on radiographs.

Reading Assignment

Pages 3-10

Objectives

Use the same objectives as listed in the textbook.

Activities

1.A, 1.B,   These may be easily performed during class time.
1.C, 1.D.

Test Questions

No test questions are necessary for this lesson.

5

CHAPTER 2
THE PRODUCTION AND PROPERTIES
OF X-RAYS

This chapter teaches students about the construction of the x-ray tube, how the x-ray tube functions to produce x-rays, and what the important properties of x-rays are for the subject of radiographic exposure. The material in this chapter can be covered in three lessons, with the test given in the fourth lesson. The material in this chapter is difficult but it is important that the students understand the material for the subsequent chapters.

LESSON 2-1: X-RAY TUBE CONSTRUCTION

Goal
Students will be able to describe the parts of a rotating anode x-ray tube.

Reading Assignment
Pages 11-13

Objectives
1. Name the 2 electrodes of the x-ray tube.
2. Describe the appearance and composition of the 2 parts of the cathode: the filament and the focusing cup.
3. Explain what the term **dual focus x-ray tube** means.
4. Describe the appearance and composition of the anode.
5. Define the term **focal track.**
6. Describe the appearance and composition of the glass housing.
7. Explain how the glass housing gets a vacuum.
8. Define the term **window.**
9. Explain the purpose of the 2 x-ray tube housings.
10. Draw a diagram of an x-ray tube and label the parts.

Activities
Activity 2.A   Homework (drawing). (Hint: It is true that the students can copy the drawings right out of the textbook, but by having

the students draw them, they will remember the lesson better.)

Test Questions

1. The negative electrode of the x-ray tube is the
    a. cathode
    b. anode

2. The 2 parts of the cathode are (pick 2)
    a. the filament   c. the focal track
    b. the window   d. the focusing cup

3. The part of the x-ray tube that surrounds the filament on three sides is the
    a. anode   c. focusing cup
    b. focal track   d. cathode

4. Which of these x-ray tube parts have tungsten in them? (list as many as apply)
    a. the anode   c. the focusing cup
    b. the filament   d. the glass envelope

5. Because the x-ray tube has 2 filaments it is called a
    a. dual focusing cup tube   c. dual anode tube
    b. dual covered tube   d. dual focus tube

6. Which of these x-ray tube parts consists of a disc that rotates when x-rays are produced?
    a. the cathode   c. the anode
    b. the filament   d. the window

7. X-rays are produced in an area around the anode called the
    a. focusing cup   c. filament
    b. focal track   d. housing

8. The glass envelope that surrounds the x-ray tube has which one of the following materials in it?

7

a. tungsten   c. lead

b. molybdenum   d. barium

9.   Which part of the x-ray tube is negatively charged?
      a. the anode   c. the filament
      b. the focal track   d. the focusing cup

10.   Which one of these has a vacuum inside it?
      a. the glass housing
      b. the metal housing

11.   After x-rays are produced they emerge through this part of the x-ray
      tube
      a. the focal track   c. the focusing cup
      b. the anode   d. the window

12.   Draw a diagram of the x-ray tube and label 5 of its parts.

Answers

1. a   4. a,b   7. b   10. a
2. a,d   5. d   8. c   11. d
3. c   6. c   9. d

LESSON 2-2: PRODUCTION OF THE X-RAY BEAM

Goal
Students will be able to describe how the x-ray tube functions to produce x-rays.

Reading Assignment
Pages 14-17

Objectives
1. List the 4 major events that produce x-rays.
2. Describe how the filament gets heated.
3. Define the terms: **incandescence, thermionic emission,** and **space charge**.
4. Explain how electrons are moved from the cathode to the anode.

8

5. Differentiate among the terms **anode, target,** and **focal spot.**
6. Explain how a small or large focal spot is produced.
7. Describe the emission of x-rays at the anode.
8. Describe the beam that is directed at the patient.
9. Explain what happens to the energy of the electrons when they are stopped at the anode.

Activities

Activity 2.B   Crossword puzzle
Activity 2.C   Placing x-ray production events in chronological order. This is a lot more challenging than it looks; it may be done as a group or individual assignment, in or out of the class period.

Test Questions

1. List the 4 major events involved in the production of x-rays.

2. When electrons are released inside the x-ray tube, they are released from the
   a. anode   c. focusing cup
   b. filament   d. window

3. Glowing of metal after heat is applied to it is called
   a. thermanescence   c. incandescence
   b. fluorescence   d. emission

4. The process of releasing electrons in the x-ray tube is called
   a. thermionic emission   c. electrolysis
   b. electromagnetism   d. induction

5. When x-rays are released during x-ray production they exist in a group called
   a. scattered radiation   c. a thermion group
   b. elements   d. the space charge

6. During x-ray production electrons travel from the
   a. cathode to the anode
   b. anode to the cathode

7. During x-ray production electrons are repelled by the _____, and attracted by the _____
   a. cathode, filament
   b. anode, cathode
   c. focusing cup, anode
   d. focal track, cathode

8. The place on the surface of the anode where the electrons are stopped is the
   a. filament
   b. target
   c. focusing cup
   d. cathode

9. The size of the area on the anode that is hit with electrons is called the
   a. target
   b. focal track
   c. focal spot
   d. bull's eye

10. If the small filament of the x-ray tube is heated during x-ray production
    a. the x-ray tube will be destroyed
    b. the glass envelope will lose its vacuum
    c. a small focal spot is produced
    d. the large filament also gets heated

11. The focal spot helps control which one of these x-ray qualities?
    a. distortion
    b. recorded detail
    c. density
    d. contrast

12. X-rays are produced at the
    a. anode
    b. filament
    c. cathode
    d. focusing cup

13. When x-rays are produced, they fly off in all directions in a spherical pattern. This phenomenon is called
    a. incandescence
    b. current
    c. thermionic emission
    d. isotropic emission

14. One purpose of the glass housing of the x-ray tube is to
    a. protect the metal housing
    b. reduce the production of x-rays

   c. absorb radiation so it doesn't leak out of the tube
   d. reduce the focal spot

15.   What percentage of the energy of the electrons is converted to
      x-rays?
      a. 1%   c. 99%
      b. 50%   d. 100%

16.   Match the part of the x-ray tube with its purpose:
      a. release electrons   1. anode
      b. repel electrons   2. glass housing
      c. stop electrons   3. filament
      d. provides a vacuum   4. focusing cup

Answers

2. b	5. d	8. b	11. b	14. c
3. c	6. a	9. c	12. a	15. a
4. a	7. c	10. c	13. d	16. a, 3 b, 4 c, 1 d, 2

LESSON 2-3: PROPERTIES OF X-RAYS

Goal
Students will be able to describe the properties of x-rays that relate to radiographic quality.

Reading Assignment
Pages 17-21

Objectives
1. Explain how x-rays travel from the anode to the patient's   body.
2. Describe the terms **photon, heterogenous,** and **polyenergetic.**
3. Describe the visibility of x-rays.
4. Describe the speed of x-rays.
5. List the 3 events that can occur when the primary beam enters the patient's body.
6. Explain how scattered radiation is produced.

7. Describe how x-rays affect radiographic film and produce an image.
8. Explain why radiographers need to be cautious about radiation protection.
9. List the properties of x-rays that are important to radiographic quality.

Activities

2.D   Word search
2.E   Chapter review

Test Questions

1.   Which of the following statements are true and which are false concerning the pattern of x-rays as they emerge from the tube and travel toward the patient's body?
a. They travel in straight lines.
b. They create a fan-shaped beam.
c. They continue to move isotropically.
d. They gather together at their point of origin.

2.   A tiny particle of energy in the x-ray beam is called a/an
a. electron   c. photon
b. thermion   d. positron

3.   Which of these words mean that x-rays have many different energies: (List all that apply.)
a. heterogenous   c. incandescent
b. thermionic   d. polyenergetic

4.   How fast do x-rays travel?
a. 86,000 miles/sec   c. 186,000 miles/sec
b. 100,000 miles/sec   d. 386,000 miles/sec

5.   The radiation that is directed toward the patient's body is called
a. remnant radiation   c. scattered radiation
b. exit radiation   d. primary radiation

6.   Are x-ray photons visible?
a. yes
b. no

7. Radiation that emerges from the patient's body and is directed toward the film is called
   a. remnant radiation
   b. exit radiation
   c. scattered radiation
   d. primary radiation

8. Radiation that is produced when x-ray photons hit the patient's body and fly off in different directions is called
   a. remnant radiation
   b. exit radiation
   c. scattered radiation
   d. primary radiation

9. Areas of a radiographic film that receive a lot of radiation will appear as what color on a radiograph?
   a. black
   b. blue
   c. white
   d. yellow

10. X-rays can cause certain materials to glow. These materials are called
    a. photons
    b. electrons
    c. phosphors
    d. atoms

11. The glowing of a material after being hit with x-rays is called
    a. incandescence
    b. fluorescence
    c. heterogenous
    d. radiation

12. Areas of a radiographic film corresponding to an area where a lot of x-ray energy was absorbed by the patient's body will appear as what color on a radiograph?
    a. black
    b. dark gray
    c. white
    d. purple

13. Radiographers must be careful about exposing the patient's body to radiation because
    a. the patient's body will become radioactive
    b. radiation can damage the patient's body
    c. the radiographer can be accused of harassment
    d. the patient can file a malpractice lawsuit

Answers

1. a-T b-F   c-T   d-F   4. c   7. b   10. c   13. b
2. c   5. d   8. c   11. b
3. a,d   6. b   9. a   12. c

SECTION II
DISTORTION

CHAPTER 3
SIZE DISTORTION

Chapter 3 begins the section on distortion with a discussion of size distortion. The student is first introduced to the distance terminology of source-image distance, object-image distance, and source-object distance. Focal-film distance and object-film distance are also defined but the book uses source-image and object-image throughout because the American Registry of Radiologic Technologists (ARRT) examination uses this terminology.

Size distortion and its effect on magnification distortion and radiographic quality is the next subject. Students are given instruction on how to calculate the image and object size, the magnification factor, and the percent of magnification with practice in activity 3.E and 3.F.

The material in this chapter can be covered in two class sessions, with the test given in the third class. This material is not too difficult unless students have a lot of trouble with math.

LESSON 3-1: SIZE DISTORTION

Goal
Students will be able to calculate distance terms and describe how to use SID and OID to control magnification.

Reading Assignment
Pages 25-31

Objectives
1. Define these terms: **source-image distance, focus-film distance, object-image distance, object-film distance, source-object distance, and focus-object distance.**
2. Given 2 of the 3 distance terms, calculate the third unknown distance.
3. Define the term **size distortion.**

15

4. Explain how the object-image distance can be used to control magnification.
5. Explain how the source-image distance can be used to control magnification.
6. State which factor, the SID or OID, has greater control over magnification.
7. Explain how to compensate for a large OID.

Activities

Activity 3.A   Calculation of distances; assign either in class or as homework.

Activity 3.B   Lab practice using the collimator light to simulate the effect of the x-ray beam on magnification.

Activity 3.C   Lab practice using x-ray exposure to see the effect of OID on magnification.

Activity 3.D   Lab practice using x-ray exposure to see the effect of SID on magnification. (Hint: Assign 3.B, 3.C, and 3.D as individual or group activities during lab times.)

Test Questions

1.   List the 2 primary factors that control the degree of size distortion.

Calculate the following:

2.   If the SID is 50 inches and the OID is 2 inches, what is the SOD?

3.   If the OID is 3 inches and the SOD is 60 inches, what is the SID?

4.   If the SID is 72 inches and the SOD is 68 inchces, what is the OID?

5.   The size of the image will be increased if
a. OID is increased
b. SID is increased
c. OID is decreased
d. the small focal spot is used instead of the large

6.   If the x-ray tube is moved from a 30 inch SID to a 60 inch SID what will occur on the image?
　　　1. The image size will increase.

16

2. The image size will decrease.
3. Magnification will decrease.
4. Magnification will increase.

a. 1 and 3   c. 2 and 3
b. 2, and 4   d. 1 and 4

7.   The most commonly used source-image distances are
       a. 72 and 50 inches   c. 60 and 40 inches
       b. 72 and 40 inches   d. 60 and 30 inches

8.   When the object is at a large distance from the film, the image can
       be made less magnified by
       a. decreasing the SOD   c. increasing the SID
       b. increasing the OID   d. decreasing the SID

9.   Which one of these is the best factor to control magnification?
       a. SID
       b. OID

Place the proper letter or letters before each statement to indicate its effect
on size distortion and magnification.
                  a. increases size distortion
                  b. decreases size distortion
                  c. increases magnification
                  d. decreases magnification

10.   Increase the OID

11.   Increase the SID

12.   Decrease the SOD while keeping the OID the same

13.   Decrease the OFD

14.   Increase the FFD

15.   Move the patient's body closer to the film

17

16. Change from a 40- to a 72-inch SID

17. Move the patient's body part 3 inches farther away from the film

18. Keep the OID at 4 inches while moving the tube from a 50- to 60-inch SID

19. Increase the OID from 2 inches to 6 inches and increase the SID from 39 to 40 inches

Answers

1. SID, OID	5. a	9. b	13. b,d	17. a,c
2. 48 inches	6. c	10. a,c	14. b,d	18. b,d
3. 63 inches	7. b	11. b,d	15. b,d	19.a,c
4. 4 inches	8. c	12. a,c	16. b,d	

LESSON 3-2: CALCULATING SIZE DISTORTION

Goal

Students will be able to calculate image and object size, the magnification factor, and the percent of magnification.

Reading Assignment

Pages 31-33

Objectives

1. Given the SID, OID, and object's size (length or width), calculate the image size (length or width).
2. Calculate the magnification factor in 2 different ways.
3. Given the magnification factor and the object size, calculate the image size.
4. Given the magnification factor and the area of the object, calculate the area of the image.
5. Given the image size and object size, calculate the percent of magnification.

Activities

Activity 3.E   Calculation of size distortion. (Hint: Assign as homework.)

Activity 3.F   Calculation of size distortion from radiographs produced during activities 3.C and 3.D. (Hint: Assign as homework or during lab time.)

Activity 3.G   Analyzing images from activity 3.C and 3.D. (Hint: Assign during lab time or class time. Students may need help with this.)

Activity 3.H   Chapter review

Test Questions

1.   If the object is 6 inches long, the SID is 72 inches, and the OID is 6 inches, how long is the image?

2.   If the object is 5 inches wide, the SID is 40 inches, and the OID is 2 inches, how wide is the image?

3.   If the image is 8 inches long, the SID is 56 inches, and the SOD is 48 inches, how long is the object?

4.   What is the magnification factor if the SID is 72 inches and the OID is 6 inches?

5.   What is the magnification factor if the SID is 40 inches and the SOD is 38 inches?

6.   What is the magnification factor if the image is 7 cm long and the object is 5 cm long?

7.   What is the magnification factor if the image is 6 inches wide and the object is 5 inches wide?

8.   If the magnification factor is 1.2 and the object length is 10 inches, what is the image length?

9.   If the object area is 6 inches by 10 inches and the magnification factor is 1.2, what is the image area?

10. What is the percent of magnification if the object is 11 inches long and the image is 14 inches long?

11. What is the percent of magnification if the object is 6 inches wide and the image is 16 inches wide?

12. If the object length is 12 inches and the image length is 24 inches, what is the magnification factor?

13. In question number 12, what is the percent of magnification?

Use these factors for questions 14-18.
object length: 7 inches
object width: 5 inches
SID: 72 inches
OID: 4 inches

14. What is the image length?

15. What is the image width?

16. What is the percent of magnification?

17. What is the magnification factor?

18. What is the area of the image?

Answers

1. 6.55	6. 1.4	11. 78%	16. 5.7%
2. 5.26	7. 1.2	12. 2	17. 1.06
3. 6.86	8. 12	13. 100%	18. 39.2
4. 1.09	9. 86.4	14. 7.41	
5. 1.05	10. 27%	15. 5.29	

CHAPTER 4
SHAPE DISTORTION

Chapter 4 ends the section on distortion with a discussion of shape distortion. First the ideal central ray-object-film alignment is analyzed. Then foreshortening is discussed, followed by elongation and spatial distortion.

This chapter can be taught in two class sessions with the third class session for the test. The material is not too difficult if students are given the opportunity to see the types of shape distortion on radiographs.

LESSON 4-1: FORESHORTENING AND ELONGATION

Goal
Students will be able to describe and use the ideal central ray-object-film relationship to avoid foreshortening and elongation.

Reading Assignment
Pages 35-42

Objectives
1. Define shape distortion and explain how it differs from size distortion.
2. List the 3 types of shape distortion.
3. Differentiate between the x-ray beam and the central ray.
4. Define the term **object**.
5. Describe the ideal relationship between the central ray, object, and film that will produce the least amount of distortion.
6. Explain how foreshortening occurs.
7. Explain how elongation occurs.
8. Explain why proper beam centering is important.

Activities
Activity 4.A   Lab activity using the collimator light to simulate shape distortion produced by poor alignment of the x-ray beam, object, and film.
Activity 4.B   Lab activity producing foreshortening on a film; requires x-ray exposure.
Activity 4.C   Lab activity producing elongation on a film; requires x-ray exposure.

21

Activity 4.D   Lab activity on proper and improper beam centering; requires x-ray exposure.

Test Questions

1.   Describe the ideal central ray-object-film relationship.

2.   Describe how foreshortening is produced.

3.   Describe how elongation is produced.

4.   Foreshortening occurs when
a. the object is angled compared with the plane of the film, and the central ray is perpendicular to the film
b. the image is longer than the object
c. the film is perpendicular to the object, and the object and beam are parallel to each other
d. the film is perpendicular to the object, and the object and beam are perpendicular to each other

5.   Elongation occurs when
a. the object is longer than the image
b. the image is longer than the object
c. the image is larger in size than the object
d. the image appears shorter than the object

6.   An image produced with the central ray at the exact center of the object will exhibit
a. more distortion at the center of the film
b. more size distortion than shape distortion
c. more distortion at the edges of the film
d. no variation in distortion over the entire film surface

7.   Which one of these is *not* a type of shape distortion?
a. foreshortening   c. elongation
b. spatial distortion   d. beam centering

8.   Which one of these types of distortion would be best at hiding a small fracture?

22

a. foreshortening

b. elongation

9.   To avoid shape distortion, place the object _____ to the film and the central ray to the object and film.
a. parallel, perpendicular
b. perpendicular, parallel

Answers

4. a	6. c	8. a
5. b	7. d	9. a

LESSON 4-2: SPATIAL DISTORTION

Goal
Students will be able to describe how spatial distortion occurs and how to avoid it.

Reading Assignment
Pages 42-44

Objectives
1. Describe superimposition.
2. Explain how spatial distortion occurs.
3. Explain the importance of the direction of the central ray when using spatial distortion to improve the image.

Activities
Activity 4.E   Lab activity producing spatial distortion; requires x-ray exposure.

Activity 4.F   Chapter review. (Hint: This can be done in class as a review before the test or, assign as homework.)

Test Questions
Use the diagram on the next page to answer questions 1-7.

23

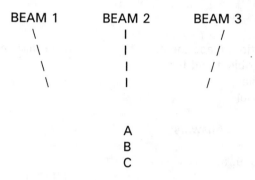

1. A radiograph produced using beam position 2 would display
   a. elongation   c. superimposition
   b. foreshortening

2. A radiograph produced using beam position 1 would display
   a. foreshortening of part A
   b. foreshortening of part C
   c. part A to the right of part C
   d. part B to the right of part A

3. A radiograph produced using beam position 3 would display
   a. superimposition of parts A, B, and C
   b. foreshortening of part B
   c. part B to the right of part C
   d. part C to the right of part A

4. A radiograph produced using beam position 1 would display foreshortening of
   a. part A   c. part C
   b. part B   d. none of the parts

5. A radiograph taken using beam position 3 would show which part on the left side of the image?
   a. part A   c. part C
   b. part B

24

6.   A radiograph taken using beam position 1 would show the most
     spatial distortion of which part?
     a. part A   c. part C
     b. part B

7.   To produce a radiograph with part A and C not superimposed which
     of these beam positions can be used? List all that apply.
     a. beam 1   c. beam 3
     b. beam 2

8.   When all the body parts in a structure are on top of each other on
     the image, this is called
     a. foreshortening   c. spatial distortion
     b. elongation   d. superimposition

9.   Spatial distortion occurs when
     a. the central ray is perpendicular to the film and the film is at an
     angle
     b. the central ray is perpendicular to the film and the object is at an
     angle
     c. the object is parallel to the film and the central ray is at an angle
     d. body parts that would normally be superimposed on the image are
     not superimposed

                                   Answers
1. c   4. d   7. a,c
2. c   5. a   8. d
3. d   6. a   9. d

                Section Review Activities on Distortion

Activity 4.G   Crossword puzzle
Activity 4.H   Word search
Activity 4.I   Multiple choice

SECTION III
THE PRIMARY EXPOSURE FACTORS

CHAPTER 5
mAs and Reciprocity

Chapter 5 is the first chapter in the section on the primary exposure factors. The radiographic quality of density is reviewed first. Then the exposure factors of milliamperage and time, and their effect on density are introduced. The three types of timers -- fractions, decimals, and milliseconds -- are analyzed, and then the students are taught how to calculate mAs.

The reciprocity law is also taught in this chapter. The book discusses the three clinical applications of the reciprocity law: control of motion, using the small focal spot, and selecting the breathing technique. Last, the student learns how to use a mAs chart.

More time is devoted to this subject in this text than in any other similar book because it is important for students to have a good foundation in primary exposure factors especially as x-ray equipment moves into the "point and shoot" era. The material in this chapter is of medium difficulty for a new student and can be taught in three class sessions with the test given in the fourth. Many practice activities accompany this chapter.

LESSON 5-1: mAs

Goal
Students will be able to describe the relationship of mAs and density and calculate mAs with any type of timer.

Reading Assignment
Pages 47-56

Objectives
1. Define the term **density.**
2. Define the term **mA,** state what it determines, and state its relationship to density.

26

3. Define the term **time,** state what it determines, and state its relationship to density.
4. Change milliseconds to a decimal or a fraction.
5. Define the term **mAs,** state what it determines, and state its relationship to density.
6. Given an mA and a time value, calculate the mAs.
7. Given 2 of the 3 factors of mA, time, or mAs, calculate the unknown factor.

Activities

Activity 5.A   Lab practice using the densitometer; use of the densitometer is required in many subsequent activities

Activity 5.B   Lab practice requiring x-ray exposure to see the effect of mA on density

Activity 5.C   Lab practice requiring x-ray exposure to see the effect of time on density

Activity 5.D   Math practice with calculation of milliseconds

Activity 5.E   Math practice with calculation of mAs

Activity 5.F   Lab practice requiring x-ray exposure to see the effect of mAs on density

Activity 5.G   Math practice with calculation of a different mAs with the same time or mA

Activity 5.H   Math practice with calculation of the unknown factor in the mAs equation

Test Questions

Do the following factors have a direct, inverse, or no relationship to density?
        a. direct
        b. inverse
        c. no relationship

1. mA   ____

2. time ____

3. mAs ____

What radiographic quality do the following factors control?
        a. density

27

      b. contrast
      c. recorded detail
      d. distortion

4. mA ____

5. time ____

6. mAs ____

7. Which one of these exposure factors determines the total quantity of x-rays produced during an exposure?
    a. mA   c. mAs
    b. time   d. Kvp

8. If the mAs is decreased by 25%, the density will be decreased by
    a. 100%   c. 50%
    b. 75%   d. 25%

9. Which one of these factors determines the amount of current in the x-ray tube when an exposure is made?
    a. mAs   c. time
    b. mA   d. none of these

10. If the mA is 200 and the time is .15, what is the mAs?
    a. 5   c. 30
    b. 24   d. 150

11. Which one of these milliseconds is the same as 1/20 sec?
    a. 5   c. 25
    b. 10   d. 50

12. Which set of factors would produce a radiograph with the greatest density?
    a. 500 mA   .10 sec   c. 500 mA   .15 sec
    b. 400 ma   .30 sec   d. 300 mA   .025 sec

13. Which set of factors would produce a radiograph with the least density?

a. 200 mA   1/30 sec   c. 300 mA   1/20 sec

b. 500 mA   3 msec   d. 600 mA   .03 sec

Calculate these mAs values:

14. 300 mA   .05 sec

15. 500 mA   2/5 sec

16. 400 mA   20 msec

17. 600 mA   .02 sec

18. 300 mA   1/3 sec

Fill in the unknown factor on this chart:

	mA	time	mAs
19.	400	.025	____
20.	200	40	____
21.	10 msec	5	____
22.	400	1/20	____

What happens to density on the radiograph with the following changes?

23. The mA is increased.

24. The time is decreased.

25. The mAs is decreased.

26. The time is doubled.

27. the mAs is cut by 25%

Answers

1. a	8. d	15. 200	22. 20
2. a	9. b	16. 8	23. density increases
3. a	10. c	17. 12	24. density decreases
4. a	11. d	18. 100	25. density decreases
5. a	12. b	19. 10	26. density doubles
6. a	13. b	20. .2	27. density decreases by 25%
7. c	14. 15	21. 500	

LESSON 5-2: RECIPROCITY

Goal
Students will be able to apply the reciprocity law to control motion, select the small focal spot, and use the breathing technique.

Reading Assignment
Pages 56-60

Objectives
1. Describe the reciprocity law.
2. Use the reciprocity law to control motion.
3. Use the reciprocity law to select the small focal spot.
4. Use the reciprocity law to use a breathing technique.

Activities
Activity 5.I   Math practice on using the reciprocity law to control motion
Activity 5.J   Math practice on using the reciprocity law to achieve a small focal spot
Activity 5.K   Math practice on using the reciprocity law to use a breathing technique

Test Questions
1.   To reduce the chance of the patient moving during the exposure, the radiographer should choose the lowest
    a. mA   c. mAs
    b. time   d. KVp

2.   Which 2 sets of mA and time are an example of the reciprocity law?
                1. 400 mA   1/20 sec
                2. 200 mA   .03 sec
                3. 500 mA   3 msec
                4. 100 mA   .20 sec

        a. 1 and 3   c. 1 and 4
        b. 2 and 4   d. 2 and 3

3.   Which one of these techniques is the best to control motion on a radiograph?

30

a. 500 mA   .01 sec   c. 100 mA 50 msec
b. 100 mA   1/20 sec   d. 200 mA .025 sec

4.   Which one of these techniques is the best for a breathing technique?
     a. 200 mA   .20 sec   c. 100 mA   400 msec
     b. 800 mA   1/20 sec   d. 25 mA   2 sec

5.   Which one of these techniques produces the best recorded detail on
     the radiograph?
     a. 400 mA   .05 sec
     b. 500 mA   .04 sec
     c. 1000 mA   20 msec
     d. 50 mA   .40 sec

Use the sample control panel from page 346 for questions
6-14 and calculate the mA and time required to achieve the mAs listed.

Calculate a breathing technique:
6. 25 mAs

7. 40 mAs

8. 12.5 mAs

Calculate the best technique to control motion:
9.   5 mAs

10. 18 mAs

11. 12 mAs

Calculate the best technique that achieves a small focal spot:
12. 4 mAs

13. 15 mAs

14. 25 mAs

Answers

1. b	6. 25 mA 1 sec	11. 1200 mA .01 sec
2. c	7. 50 mA 4/5 sec	12. 200 mA .02 sec
3. a	8. 25 mA .5 sec	13. 100 mA .15 sec
4. d	9. 1000 mA .005 sec	14. 200 mA 125 msec
5. d	10. 1200 mA .015 sec	

LESSON 5-3: mAs CHARTS

Goal
Students will be able to use a mAs chart.

Reading Assignment
Pages 60-62

Objective
1. Use an mAs chart to find the mA, time, or mAs.

Activities
Activity 5.L   Practice using an mAs chart; spend time during class with this.

Activity 5.M   Chapter review

Test Questions
Use the mAs chart on page 61 to find the answers for questions 1-10.

Find the mAs:
1.   300 mA 20 msec

2.   600 mA .025 sec

3.   100 mA 1/15 sec

4.   50 mA .015 sec

Find the mA:

5.   9 mAs 15 msec

32

6.   12 mAs .03 sec

7.   5 mAs 1/20 sec

Find the time in any unit:

8.   3 mAs 100 mA

9.   7.5 mAs 300 mA

10.   .50 mAs 25 mA

                                    Answers
1. 6mAs   4. .75 mAs   7. 100 mA   10. .02 sec
2. 15 mAs   5. 600 mA   8. .03
3. 6.66 mAs   6. 400 mA   9. 25 msec,1/40 sec,.025 sec

CHAPTER 6
THE INVERSE SQUARE LAW

Chapter 6 introduces the student to the effect of distance changes on beam intensity using the inverse square law. This concept is expanded by analyzing the effect of distance changes on density using the density maintenance formula.

The material in this chapter can be covered in two classes with a test given in the third session. The concepts are not too difficult, but the math can be a stumbling block.

LESSON 6-1: THE INVERSE SQUARE LAW

Goal
Students will understand how the intensity of radiation changes when the SID changes, and be able to calculate the change in intensity.

Reading Assignment
Pages 63-67

Objectives
1. Describe what happens to the radiation intensity at the film as the distance between the x-ray tube and film is increased or decreased.
2. State the inverse square law and its formula.
3. Use the inverse square law formula to calculate the new radiation intensity when the SID is increased or decreased.
4. Use the inverse square law rule of thumb to calculate the new radiation intensity when the SID is doubled or cut in half.
5. Estimate the new radiation intensity when the distance between the x-ray tube and film is increased or decreased.
6. Explain what happens to the density on a radiograph when the SID is increased or decreased.
7. Explain how radiation intensity is measured.

Activities
Activity 6.A   Using the collimator light beam to simulate the change in beam intensity with distance changes

Activity 6.B   Math practice with the inverse square law formula
Activity 6.C   Math practice with the inverse square law rule of thumb
Activity 6.D   Lab practice on the inverse square law requiring x-ray
exposure and intensity measurement with an ionization
chamber

Test Questions

1.   If the x-ray tube is moved farther away from the film, the radiation
intensity at the film
a. increases
b. decreases

2.   If the x-ray tube is moved closer to the film, the collimator light will
a. cover a smaller area of the film
b. cover a larger area of the film

3.   If the distance between the x-ray tube and the film is cut in half, the
radiation intensity at the film
a. is cut in half
b. quadruples
c. is reduced by four times

Calculate the new radiation intensity for questions 4-10.

	I_1	D_1	D_2
4.	30 mR	72 inches	36 inches
5.	20 mR	40 inches	80 inches
6.	10 mR	72 inches	40 inches
7.	60 mR	56 inches	40 inches
8.	12 mR	40 inches	60 inches
9.	15 mR	44 inches	58 inches
10.	120 mR	72 inches	56 inches

Answers

1. b	5. 5 mR	9. 8.6 mR
2. a	6. 32 mR	10. 198.4 mR
3. b	7. 117 mR	
4. 120 mR	8. 5.3 mR	

LESSON 6-2: THE DENSITY MAINTENANCE FORMULA

Goal

Students will be able to apply the density maintenance formula.

Reading Assignment

Pages 67-72

Objectives

1. State the density maintenance formula.
2. Use the density maintenance formula to calculate the new mAs when the SID is increased or decreased.
3. Use the density maintenance formula rule of thumb to calculate the new mAs, which will maintain film density when the SID is doubled or cut in half.
4. Use the density maintenance formula to calculate the new time when the SID is increased or decreased.
5. Estimate the new mAs when the SID is increased or decreased.

Activities

Activity 6.E   Math practice with the density maintenance formula

Activity 6.F   Lab practice on the density maintenance formula
                     x-ray exposure

Activity 6.G   Math practice calculating the new time with the density maintenance formula

Activity 6.H   Math practice with the density maintenance formula rule of thumb

Activity 6.I   Practice estimating the new mAs with distance changes

Activity 6.J   Chapter review

Test Questions

1.   Use of the density maintenance formula tells the radiographer
   a. the new beam intensity at the film when the SID changes
   b. the new mAs to use to maintain density when the SID changes
   c. how to adjust the collimation when the SID changes

36

d. the new radiation dose the patient will receive when the SID changes

2.	If the same exposure factors are used on 4 different radiographs taken with the 4 SIDs listed below, which radiograph would display the least density? The one taken at
a. 34-inch SID			c. 60-inch SID
b. 40-inch SID			d. 72-inch SID

3.	When adjusting the exposure factors after calculating the density maintenance formula, which one of these factors is usually the best to change?
a. mA				c. SID
b. exposure time			d. Kvp

4.	If the original mAs is 15 and the SID changes from 40 inches to 62 inches, which one of these mAs values would produce a radiograph with density the same as the original radiograph taken at 15 mAs?
a. 6.2 mAs			c. 36 mAs
b. 15 mAs			d. 52.4 mAs

Radiograph A	Radiograph B
600 mA	400 mA
.05 sec	.15 sec
36-inch SID	72-inch SID

5.	Using the above exposure factors, which one of these statements is true about the 2 different radiographs?
a. radiograph A would display more density than radiograph B
b. radiograph A would display less density than radiograph B
c. radiograph B would display less density than radiograph A
d. the 2 radiographs would display the same density

Calculate the new mAs for questions 6-10.

	old mAs	D_1	D_2
6.	25 mAs	64 inches	36 inches
7.	12 mAs	40 inches	80 inches

37

8.	15 mAs	72 inches	36 inches
9.	50 mAs	40 inches	50 inches
10.	40 mAs	44 inches	36 inches

Answers

1. b	6.	7.9 mAs
2. d	7.	48 mAs
3. b	8.	3.75 mAs
4. c	9.	78 mAs
5. c	10.	26.7 mAs

CHAPTER 7
RADIOGRAPHIC CONTRAST

Chapter 7 expands on the quality factor of contrast. The chapter begins with the concepts of high and low contrast and short and long scale contrast. Then subject contrast is analyzed through tissue density, differential absorption, tissue thickness, muscle tone, fat content, water retention, and the use of contrast media to alter radiographic contrast.

The exposure factor of kVp is the next subject. How high and low kVp techniques alter the energy and penetrating ability of the beam is first analyzed followed by the effect of kVp on scattered radiation production and radiographic contrast.

The material in chapter seven is sometimes difficult for students to understand. The content can be covered in two class sessions with a test given in the third session, but if students are having difficulty with the material, perhaps a review session before the test would be helpful.

LESSON 7-1: RADIOGRAPHIC CONTRAST

Goal
Students will understand the concepts of high and low contrast, short and long scale contrast, and subject contrast.

Reading Assignment
Pages 73-80

Objectives
1. Define contrast.
2. Differentiate between high and low contrast.
3. Differentiate between short and long scale contrast.
4. Define subject contrast.
5. Explain how tissue density affects subject contrast and the appearance of the image on the radiograph.
6. Define the term differential absorption.
7. Explain how tissue thickness affects subject contrast and the appearance of the image on the radiograph.
8. Describe how muscle tone, fat content, and water retention affect radiographic contrast.

9.   Describe how contrast media is used to alter radiographic contrast.

Activities

Activity 7.A   A short drawing activity

Activity 7.B   Lab activity requiring x-ray exposure to show the effect of water retention on scattered radiation.

Test Questions

1.   Write the definition of radiographic contrast.

2.   Which type of image would be considered a low contrast image?
a. black and white and few gray shades
b. black, white, and many gray shades

3.   Which one of these has the least tissue density?
a. air   c. fat
b. muscle   d. bone

4.   Which one of these body components would display the least radiographic density?
a. air   c. fat
b. muscle   d. bone

5.   The ability of the patient's body to absorb radiation differently depending on the tissue density of its components is called
a. high contrast   c. attenuation
b. differential absorption   d. short scale contrast

6.   Which would absorb the least amount of radiation?
a. a body part with many electrons
b. a body part with few electrons

7.   Which one of these body parts composed of identical matter would absorb the least amount of radiation?
a. a thick body component
b. a thin body component

40

8. Which one of these body parts composed of identical matter would display the most radiographic density?
   a. a thick body component
   b. a thin body component

9. Radiographs of which one of these patients would display short scale contrast?
   a. a patient who has been bedridden for a long time
   b. a patient with a disease that has demineralized his bones
   c. a patient who has retained water due to disease
   d. a patient who has a muscular physique

10. Which one of these contrast materials will appear black on a radiograph?
    a. air   c. iodine
    b. barium

11. Short scale contrast is also called
    a. high contrast
    b. low contrast

12. Which one of these contrast media is most appropriate for use in the gallbladder?
    a. air   c. iodine
    b. barium

Answers

2. b	4. d	6. b	8. b	10. a	12. c
3. a	5. b	7. b	9. d	11. a	

LESSON 7-2: KILOVOLTAGE (kVp)

Goal
Students will understand how kVp affects contrast.

Reading Assignment
Pages 81-86

Objectives

1. Explain how kVp determines the energy of the photons in a beam.
2. Describe the effect of high and low kVp techniques on the average energy of the beam, penetrating ability, differential absorption, the type of contrast produced, and the scale of contrast produced.
3. Describe the effect of fog on the image.
4. Explain how changing the kVp can change the amount of scattered radiation produced.
5. Define the term **attenuation**.

Activities

Activity 7.C   Lab activity requiring x-ray exposure to analyze the production of scattered radiation by the patient

Activity 7.D   Chapter review

Test Questions

1. A high energy photon will probably be produced by an electron traveling from the cathode to the anode with
   a. a lot of energy
   b. only a little energy

2. A photon produced with high kVp would be most likely to
   a. penetrate through body tissues
   b. be absorbed by body tissues

3. A radiographic image with a lot of fog would demonstrate
   a. high radiographic contrast
   b. low radiographic contrast

4. More scattered radiation is produced by a
   a. high kVp beam
   b. low kVp beam

5. kVp is the controlling factor for
   a. density   c. recorded detail
   b. contrast   d. distortion

6. Which increases differential absorption?
a. a high kVp beam
b. a low kVp beam

7. A photon which has changed its direction and lost energy is what type of a photon?
a. primary   c. scattered
b. absorbed   d. attenuated

8. Which one of these is the term toi describe the reduction of radiation as it passes through matter?
a. differential absorption   c. subject contrast
b. radiographic contrast   d. attenuation

9. Where does most scattered radiation originate?
a. at the cathode
b. in the x-ray tabletop
c. in the patient
d. in the lead wall barriers

10. What effect does scattered radiation have on a radiographic image? List all that apply.
a. it increases density
b. it increases contrast
c. it decreases density
d. it decreases contrast

Answers

1. a	4. a	7. c	10. a, d
2. a	5. b	8. d	
3. b	6. b	9. c	

CHAPTER 8
mAs AND kVp RELATIONSHIP

Chapter 8 explains the relationship between mAs and kVp beginning with the subject of selecting optimum kVp to ensure penetration of the body part, sufficient radiographic contrast, and a predictable amount of scattered radiation. Then the fact that mAs is the controlling factor for density and that kVp is the controlling factor for contrast, but also affects density, is reinforced. The last part of the chapter teaches the student how to use the 15% rule to control contrast and motion.

This material does not seem too difficult to instructors, but it is sometimes difficult for students to understand, and more importantly, to remember and to use in clinical situations. The chapter can be divided into two class sessions with the test given in the third session.

LESSON 8-1: mAs AND kVp RELATIONSHIP

Goal
Students will be able to select optimum kVp and describe the relationship between mAs and kVp.

Reading Assignment
Pages 87-92

Objectives
1. Define optimum kVp.
2. Explain why optimum kVp will always penetrate the part, produce sufficient contrast, and produce an acceptable amount of scattered radiation.
3. List the optimum kVp for common body parts.
4. Explain how mAs and kVp control the quantity and quality of the beam.
5. Describe how mAs and kVp control density and contrast.

Activities
Activity 8.A   Requires students to list the kVp used for common body parts in their clinical assignments

44

Test Questions

1.   Write the controlling factor for density.

2.   Write the controlling factor for contrast.

Use the following statements to answer questions 3-6. List all that apply.
    a. density increases   d. contrast decreases
    b. contrast increases   e. density stays the same
    c. density decreases   f. contrast stays the same

3.   The original radiograph is of good quality and the mAs is increased.

4.   The original radiograph is of good quality and the kVp is increased.

5.   The original radiograph is of good quality and the mAs is decreased
        and the kVp is decreased.

6.   The original radiograph is of good quality and the kVp is decreased.

For questions 7-9, write the optimum kVp for the body part listed.
7.   abdomen without barium

8.   spine

9.   ribs

For questions 10-12, explain what an increase in kVp would do to

10.   the average energy of the photons in the beam

11.   the amount of scattered radiation produced

12.   the penetration of the body part

True or False
13.   kVp controls density.

45

14. mAs determines the quantity of radiation in the beam.

15. mAs affects contrast.

16. kVp determines the quality of radiation in the beam.

17. mAs controls density.

18. kVp affects density.

19. Optimum kVp will always penetrate the body part.

20. Optimum kVp should be used to control density.

Answers

1. mAs	5. b, c	9. 70	16. T	20. F
2. kVp	6. b, c	13. F	17. T	
3. a, f	7. 70	14. T	18. T	
4. a, d	8. 80	15. F	19. T	

LESSON 8-2: THE 15% RULE

Goal
Students will be able to apply the 15% rule.

Reading Assignment
Pages 92-97

Objectives
1. Explain the purpose of the 15% rule.
2. Perform calculations of the 15% rule.
3. Use the 15% rule to change contrast.
4. Use the 15% rule to control motion.
5. Explain the limitation on the 15% rule imposed by exposure latitude.
6. Apply the 15% rule in the 60-90 kVp range.

Activities

Activity 8.B   Math practice with the 15% rule
Activity 8.C   Math practice using the 15% rule to control motion and
                contrast
Activity 8.D   Lab activity requiring x-ray exposure showing
                the results of the 15% rule
Activity 8.E   Math practice with the 15% rule in the 60-90 kVp range
Activity 8.F   Chapter review

Test Questions

Use the following statements to answer questions 1-4. List all that apply.

a. density increases   d. contrast decreases
b. contrast increases   e. density stays the same
c. density decreases   f. contrast stays the same

1.   The original radiograph is of good quality, the kVp is increased, and
      the mAs is decreased according to the 15% rule.

2.   The original radiograph is of good quality, the kVp is decreased, and
      the mAs is increased according to the 15% rule.

3.   The original exposure factors are 10 mAs and 80 kVp. The technique
      is changed to 5 mAs and 90 kVp.

4.   The original exposure factors are 7 mAs and 75 kVp. The technique
      is changed to 14 mAs and 60 kVp.

Using the 15% rule calculate the new kVp with the change in the mAs.

original mAs	original kVp	new mAs	new kVp
5. 20	80	10	____
6. 8	70	4	____
7. 15	90	30	____
8. 12	75	6	____
9. 4	100	8	____

Using the 15% rule, calculate the new mAs with the change in the kVp.

original mAs	original kVp	new mAs	new kVp
10. 18	85	___	75
11. 25	100	___	115
12. 3	70	___	80
13. 6	90	___	80
14. 50	80	___	70

Answers

1. d, e	5. 90 kVp	9. 85 kVp	13. 12 mAs
2. b, e	6. 80 kVp	10. 36 mAs	14. 100 mAs
3. d, e	7. 80 kVp	11. 12.5 mAs	
4. b, c	8. 85 kVp	12. 1.5 mAs	

Section Review Activities on the Primary Exposure Factors

Activity 8.G   Multiple choice and math questions
Activity 8.H   Word search
Activity 8.I   Crossword puzzle

SECTION IV
CONTROL OF SCATTERED RADIATION

CHAPTER 9
GRIDS AND THE BUCKY

Chapter 9 begins the section dealing with control of scattered radiation. Chapter 9 itself begins with a review of the characteristics of scattered radiation and then instructs students on grid construction and use. Mention is made of the parallel and crossed grid types, but most of the chapter deals with the focused grid because that is the most popular type.

The material in this chapter will require three class sessions with the test given in the fourth. The subject matter is not too difficult for students to understand.

LESSON 9-1: GRID CONSTRUCTION

Goal
Students will be able to describe the construction of a parallel, crossed, and focused grid

Reading Assignment
Pages 101-107

Objectives
1. Compare the energy and direction of scattered radiation with primary radiation.
2. Describe the effect of scattered radiation on density and contrast.
3. Give the name of the man who invented the grid and the date he did so.
4. Explain the purpose of using a grid.
5. Describe these aspects of grid construction: the strips, interspaces, covering, face, and edge.
6. Describe the construction of a focused grid and explain why it is the most common grid in use.
7. Describe the construction and limitations of parallel and crossed grids.
8. Define the term **grid ratio** and list the most common ratios.

49

9.   Given a grid strip and interspace measurement, calculate the grid ratio.
10. State the advantage of a high ratio grid.
11. Define the term **grid frequency**.

Activities

Activity 9.A   A brief drawing assignment of the edge and face of the three grid types

Test Questions

True or False
1.   Scattered radiation is produced at the anode of the x-ray tube.

2.   Scattered radiation travels in a different direction from primary radiation.

3.   Scattered radiation increases fog and decreases radiographic contrast.

4.   Scattered radiation puts density on the film.

5.   Scattered radiation has more energy than primary radiation.

For questions 6-9, indicate whether the statements below describe a crossed, parallel or focused grid.
   C = crossed
   P = parallel
   F = focused

6.   This type will clean up the most scattered radiation.
7.   The grid strips are always placed parallel to each other.

8.   Pattern of strips matches the way the x-ray beam emerges from the tube.

9.   This type has the most restrictive pattern for angling the central ray.

10. This type has a grid focusing distance.

11.   A grid which has strips that are .060 inches high and interspaces
that are .010 inches wide has a
a. 60:1 grid ratio   c. 6:1 grid ratio
b. 12:1 grid ratio   d. .60:1 grid ratio

12.   Which of these is the purpose of the grid? List all that apply.
a. prevent scattered radiation from reaching the film
b. prevent primary radiation from reaching the film
c. absorb primary radiation
d. absorb scattered radiation

13.   Grid ratio is
a. the width of the lead strips compared to the width of the spaces
between them
b. the height of the lead strips compared to the distance between
the strips
c. the height of the lead strips compared to the height of the
interspaces
d. the height of the grid multiplied by its width

14.   Which one of these grid ratios will clean up the most scattered
radiation?
a. 6:1   c. 12:1
b. 8:1   d. 16:1

15.   The number of grid lines in an inch defines
a. grid focusing distance
b. grid focal range
c. grid frequency
d. grid cut-off

16.   The acceptable range of source-image distances that can be used
with a focused grid is determined by the
a. grid focusing distance
b. grid ratio
c. grid frequency
d. focal spot

Answers

1. F	5. F	9. C	13. b
2. T	6. C	10. F	14. d
3. T	7. P	11. C	5. c
4. T	8. F	12. a, d	16. a

LESSON 9-2: GRID CUT-OFF

Goal

Students will be able to avoid grid cut-off.

Reading Assignment

Pages 107-112

Objectives

1. Define the term **grid cut-off.**
2. List 5 ways in which grid cut-off can occur.
3. Describe the grid focusing distance and explain how it determines the focal range.
4. Explain how to angle the tube in order to avoid grid cut-off.
5. Explain how to center the x-ray beam to the grid to avoid grid cut-off.
6. Explain how using the grid upside down can cause grid cut-off.
7. Give the name of the man who invented the Bucky and the date he did so.
8. Describe the function of the Bucky device.

Activities

Activity 9.B   Lab requiring x-ray exposure to demonstrate the effect of SID on grid cut-off

Activity 9.C   Lab requiring x-ray exposure to demonstrate the effect of tube angle on grid cut-off

Activity 9.D   Lab requiring x-ray exposure to demonstrate the effect of grid angle on grid cut-off

Activity 9.E   Lab requiring x-ray exposure to demonstrate the effect of beam centering on grid cut-off

Activity 9.F   Lab requiring x-ray exposure to demonstrate the effect of using the grid upside down on grid cut-off

Activity 9.G   Requires student to list whether a grid is used for common exams

Test Questions

1.   Write the definition of the term **grid cut-off.**

For questions 2-6, indicate whether the maneuver will cause grid cut-off with a focused grid.
       Y = Yes, it will cause grid cut-off.
       N = No, it will not cause grid cut-off.

2.   Using a SID below the focal range.

3.   Angling the central ray in the same direction as the center line of the grid.

4.   Moving the central ray 4 inches to the side of the center line of the grid.

5.   Placing the grid so its center line points toward the film.

6.   Placing the grid so its face is perpendicular to the central ray.

7.   Using a SID in the middle of the focal range.

8.   Grid cut-off occurs when
       a. scattered radiation is absorbed by the grid
       b. primary radiation is absorbed by the grid
       c. scattered radiation gets through the grid
       d. primary radiation gets through the grid

9.   Who invented the Bucky?
       a. Wilhelm Conrad Roentgen   c. Hollis Potter
       b. Ed Jerman   d. Gustave Bucky

10.   The purpose of the Bucky is to
       a. improve the recorded detail of the grid lines
       b. increase grid ratio

c. blur grid lines
d. increase grid frequency

Answers

2. Y	5. Y	8. b
3. N	6. N	9. c
4. Y	7. N	10. c

LESSON 9-3: GRID SELECTION

Goal

Students will be able to decide when to use a grid.They will be able to compensate with mAs for a grid ratio change.

Reading Assignment

Pages 112-114

Objectives

1. Explain how it is decided when to use a grid, what pattern, and what grid ratio to use.
2. Describe the effect on density when a grid is used or changed.
3. Calculate the new mAs to be used when changing from non-grid to a grid or when changing grid ratios.

Activities

Activity 9.H Math practice calculating the new mAs when the grid ratio is changed

Activity 9.I Lab requiring x-ray exposure to analyze the effect of grid ratio on density

Activity 9.J Chapter review

Test Questions

For questions 1-8, indicate whether or not a grid should be used.

Y = Yes, a grid should be used.
N = No, a grid should not be used.

1. The body part measures 22 cm.

2.   60 kVp is used.

3.   An increase in contrast is required.

4.   A hand exam is being performed.

5.   An abdominal exam is being performed.

6.   A skull exam is being performed.

7.   80 kVp is being used.

8.   The body part measures 8 cm.

Calculate the new mAs to be used with the following grid ratio changes:

original mAs	original grid	new grid	new mAs
9. 10	8:1	16:1	___
10. 18	12:1	6:1	___
11. 7	16:1	8:1	___
12.1.5	5:1	12:1	___
13. 30	16:1	12:1	___

Answers

1. Y	5. Y	9. 15 mAs	13. 25 mAs
2. N	6. Y	10. 10.8 mAs	
3. Y	7. Y	11. 4.7 mAs	
4. N	8. N	12. 3.75 mAs	

CHAPTER 10
METHODS TO CONTROL SCATTER

Chapter 10 continues the discussion of control of scattered radiation beginning with the subject of beam restriction. Very brief mention is made of diaphragms and cones, but the main topic is the collimator. The next topic is filtration. Although the main purpose of filtration is to reduce the patient's radiation dose, filtration does alter the characteristics of the beam and affects density, contrast, and the amount of scattered radiation produced. The chapter ends with a variety of miscellaneous methods to control scatter including the air-gap technique, use of a lead blocker, compression, and using some cassettes backwards.

The material is easily divided into three class sessions with the test given in the fourth class period. Students usually understand this material without much difficulty.

LESSON 10-1: BEAM RESTRICTION

Goal
Students will be able to describe the effect of collimation of the beam on density, and contrast.

Reading Assignment
Pages 115-119

Objectives
1. Describe the two advantages of restricting the beam.
2. Describe the operation of the lead shutters in the collimator.
3. Explain how automatic collimation works.
4. Describe how the light field and light localizer are obtained.
5. Explain the effect of collimation on the amount of scattered radiation produced at the patient's body.
6. Describe the effect of collimation on density and contrast.
7. Calculate the new mAs to be used when the collimation field size is changed.

Activities

Activity 10.A   Math practice with technique compensation when changing the collimation field size

Activity 10.B   Lab requiring x-ray exposure to analyze the effects of changing collimation field size

Test Questions

1. A patient with a large abdomen would produce
   a. more scattered radiation than a patient with a small abdomen
   b. less scattered radiation than a patient with a small abdomen
   c. the same amount of scattered radiation as a patient with a small abdomen

2. The function of the lead shutters in the collimator is to
   a. increase density and decrease contrast
   b. absorb scattered radiation after it is produced in the patient's body
   c. absorb the primary radiation at the edges of the beam
   d. allow primary radiation through and absorb scattered radiation

3. Changing the collimation field size from 14X17 to10X12 will have what effect on density?
   a. increases it
   b. decreases it

4. Changing the collimation field size from 14X17 to 10X12 will have what effect on contrast?
   a. increases it
   b. decreases it

5. Changing the collimation field size from 14X17 to 10 X 12 will have what effect on scattered radiation production?
   a. increases it
   b. decreases it

6. Changing the collimation field size from 14 X 17 to 10 X 12 will have what effect on the patient's radiation dose?

a. increases it
b. decreases it

7.   The field light of a collimator is obtained from
        a. the light resulting from x-ray production
        b. a light bulb and a mirror
        c. a sensor in the Bucky tray
        d. reducing the field size

8.   Automatic collimation is produced by
        a. changing the angle of the mirror in the collimator
        b. the light bulb in the collimator
        c. a sensor in the Bucky tray
        d. the phototimer

Calculate the new mAs required to maintain density when the collimation field size is changed.

original mAs	original	new field size	new mAs size
9. 10	8X10	14X17	____
10. 7	10X12	14X17	____
11.40	14X17	8X10	____
12. 14	14X17	10X12	____
13. 1.25	10X12	8X10	____

Answers

1. a	5. b	9. 7.1	13. 1.4
2. c	6. b	10. 5.6	
3. b	7. b	11. 56	
4. a	8. c	12. 17.5	

LESSON 10-2: FILTRATION

Goal

        Students will understand the purpose and principles of filtration and be able to use a compensatory filter.

Reading Assignment

Pages 119-123

Objectives

1. Explain the main purpose of filtration.
2. Describe the effect filtration has on the energy of the photons in the beam.
3. Describe the effect filtration has on density and contrast.
4. Explain how inherent filtration is achieved.
5. Describe the appearance and placement of added filtration.
6. State the amount of filtration necessary for an x-ray tube operating at over 70 kVp.
7. State the purpose of using a compensatory filter.
8. Explain how to use wedges and trough compensatory filters.

Activities

Activity 10.C   Lab requiring x-ray exposure to demonstrate the effect of compensatory filters

Test Questions

1. Which one of these types of filters is sometimes shaped like a trough?
   a. inherent filtration
   b. added filtration
   c. total filtration
   d. compensatory filtration

2. A decrease in filtration has what effect on density?
   a. increases it
   b. decreases it

3. A decrease in filtration has what effect on contrast?
   a. increases it
   b. decreases it

4. A decrease in filtration has what effect on scattered radiation production?
   a. increases it
   b. decreases it

5.   A decrease in filtration has what effect on the energy of the photons in the beam?
     a. increases it
     b. decreases it

6.   The window of the x-ray tube produces which type of filtration?
     a. inherent   c. added
     b. total   d. compensatory

7.   If a radiograph of an AP thoracic spine is taken with a wedge compensatory filter, where should the thin end of the filter be placed?
     a. over the superior aspect of the spine
     b. over the inferior aspect of the spine

8.   A radiographer can remove which of these filters? Write all letters that apply.
     a. inherent   c. added
     b. total   d. compensatory

9.   Which one of these exams is most appropriate for using a trough compensatory filter?
     a. lateral lumbar spine   c. postanterior chest
     b. lateral skull   d. kidney-ureter bladder

10. Density is made more equal on the image by which type of filter?
     a. inherent   c. added
     b. total   d. compensatory

11. The amount of total filtration required for x-ray tubes operated at over 70 kVp is
     a. .25 mm aluminum equivalent
     b. .5 mm aluminum equivalent
     c. 2.0 mm aluminum equivalent
     d. 2.5 mm aluminum equivalent

12. What material usually is used to make an added filter?

a. tungsten   c. lead

b. aluminum   d. molybdenum

Answers

1. d	4. b	7. b	10. d
2. a	5. b	8. d	11. d
3. a	6. a	9. c	12. b

LESSON 10-3: MISCELLANEOUS METHODS TO CONTROL SCATTER

Goal

Students will have a basic understanding of how scattered radiation is controlled by the air-gap technique, lead blockers, compression, and the back of a cassette.

Reading Assignment

Pages 123-126

Objectives

1. Describe how an air-gap is achieved.
2. Explain how using an air-gap affects density and contrast.
3. Describe how to use a lead blocker.
4. Explain the effect of a lead blocker on density and contrast.
5. Describe how to use compression to change the amount of scattered radiation produced.
6. Explain how using compression changes density and contrast.
7. Explain how using certain cassettes backwards changes density and contrast.

Activities

Activity 10.D   Lab requiring x-ray exposure to demonstrate the effect of the air-gap technique

Activity 10.E   Lab requiring x-ray exposure to demonstrate the effect of lead blockers

Activity 10.F   Chapter review

Test Questions

Indicate which one the statement is referring to:

A = air-gap
B = lead blocker
C = compression
D = using the cassette backwards

1. Acts like a filter.

2. Requires a long OID.

3. Used best on abdominal exams.

4. Used on lateral sacral and coccygeal exams.

5. Requires a long SID.

6. Used most often on a posteranterior chest exam.

7. Requires the application of the density maintenance formula.

8. Used when there is a large area of unabsorbed primary radiation.

9. The patient lies prone.

10. Used often during an IVP exam.

Answers

1. D	4. B	7. A	10. C
2. A	5. A	8. B	
3. C	6. A	9. C	

SECTION V
RECORDED DETAIL

CHAPTER 11
GEOMETRIC FACTORS
AFFECTING RECORDED DETAIL

Chapter 11 begins the section on the radiographic quality of recorded detail. The geometric factors of the focal spot, OID, and SID that affect recorded detail are analyzed in this chapter. Chapters 12 and 13 discuss the material factors of film and intensifying screens.

The chapter begins by defining recorded detail and differentiating recorded detail from visibility of detail. How recorded detail is measured is the next subject; then the geometric factors are analyzed beginning with the focal spot size, then OID, and then SID. The chapter ends with instruction on the calculation of unsharpness.

The material is easily divided into three class sessions with the test given in the fourth class period. Students usually understand this material easily but have difficulty seeing differences in recorded detail on radiographs. Slight differences in recorded detail disappear when images are transposed to a text book so images are not included in this chapter. Instructors should take time in each class session to show students radiographs.

LESSON 11-1: INTRODUCTION TO RECORDED DETAIL

Goal
Students will be able to describe the quality factor of recorded detail and recognize it on a radiograph.

Reading Assignment
Pages 129-133

Objectives
1.   Define the term **recorded detail**.
2.   Differentiate between recorded detail and visibility of detail.

63

3. List the 7 factors that affect recorded detail.
4. Describe how a resolution grid is used to measure recorded detail.
5. Differentiate among the terms **penumbra, edge gradient,** and **unsharpness.**
6. Recognize differences in recorded detail on radiographs.

Activities
No activities accompany this lesson.

Test Questions
1. Write the definition of recorded detail.

2. List the 7 factors that affect recorded detail.

3. A resolution grid is a
    a. device to reduce scattered radiation
    b. test tool to measure recorded detail
    c. device use to adjust the size of the beam
    d. device used to measure the size of the focal spot

4. A line pair of a resolution grid is
    a. a pair of two metal lines
    b. two metal lines and the two spaces around them
    c. one metal line and the space adjacent to it
    d. an imaginary device created by a computer

5. The overall quality of the finished radiograph is
    a. recorded detail
    b. visibility of detail

6. The ability of an imaging system to record two adjacent structures as separate structures defines
    a. resolution   c. unsharpness
    b. edge gradient   d. penumbra

7. As unsharpness increases, recorded detail
    a. increases
    b. decreases

64

Answers

3. b   5. b   7.b
4. c   6. a

LESSON 11-2: GEOMETRIC FACTORS
AFFECTING RECORDED DETAIL

Goal
Students will understand how the focal spot, OID, and SID affect recorded detail.

Reading Assignment
Pages 133-137

Objectives
1. List the geometric factors that affect recorded detail.
2. Explain how a change in the focal spot affects recorded detail.
3. Explain how a change in OID affects recorded detail.
4. Explain how a change in SID affects recorded detail.
5. Describe how changes in OID and SID can affect both recorded detail and distortion.

Activities
Activity 11.A   Lab requiring x-ray exposure to demonstrate the effect on recorded detail when the focal spot is changed
Activity 11.B   Lab requiring x-ray exposure to demonstrate the effect on recorded detail when OID is changed
Activity 11.C   Lab requiring x-ray exposure to demonstrate the effect on recorded detail when SID is changed

Test Questions
1. List the geometric factors that affect recorded detail.

2. Increasing the SID and adjusting the exposure factors with the density maintenance formula will
   a. reduce the object-image distance

    b. increase recorded detail
    c. increase unsharpness
    d. reduce density

3.   If the small focal spot is used instead of the large focal spot
    a. contrast will increase
    b. recorded detail will increase
    c. unsharpness will increase
    d. density will increase

4.   Which one of the following combinations of factors will produce an image with the best recorded detail?
    a. small focal spot, long SID, short OID
    b. large focal spot, long SID, long OID
    c. small focal spot, short SID, long OID
    d. large focal spot, long SID, short OID

5.   Which one of the following will produce the most improvement in recorded detail?
    a. a change to the small focal spot
    b. an increase in the SID
    c. a decrease in the OID

6.   An increase in SID will
    a. increase magnification and decrease recorded detail
    b. decrease magnification and decrease recorded detail
    c. increase magnification and increase recorded detail
    d. decrease magnification and increase recorded detail

7.   An increase in OID will
    a. increase magnification and decrease recorded detail
    b. decrease magnification and decrease recorded detail
    c. increase magnification and increase recorded detail
    d. decrease magnification and increase recorded detail

Indicate whether the following statements will increase, decrease, or have no effect on recorded detail.
    I = increase

D = decrease
N = no effect

8.　　The OID is changed from 2 inches to 6 inches.

9.　　The focal spot is changed from .6 mm to 2.0 mm.

10.　　The mAs is changed from 1.75 to 2.25.

11.　　The SID is changed from 40 inches to 72 inches.

12.　　The collimation field size is changed from 8 X 10 to 14 X 17.

13.　　The OID is changed from 8 inches to 6 inches.

14.　　The kVp is changed from 80 to 70.

Answers

2. b	5. c	8. D	11. I	14. N
3. b	6. d	9. D	12. N	
4. a	7. a	10. N	13. I	

LESSON 11-3: CALCULATION OF UNSHARPNESS

Goal
Students will be able to calculate the amount of unsharpness.

Reading Assignment
Pages 137-138

Objectives
1.　Write the formula for calculating unsharpness.
2.　Given the focal spot size, OID, and either the SID or SOD, calculate the amount of unsharpness.

Activities
Activity 11.D　Math practice on calculating unsharpness

Activity 11.E   Math practice on calculating unsharpness using the
                radiographs from Activities 11.A,11.B, and 11.C
Activity 11.F   Chapter review

Test Questions

Use the factors below to answer questions 1-4:
        focal spot = .6 mm
        OID = 6 inches
        SID = 72 inches

1.   Calculate the amount of unsharpness.

2.   Calculate the amount of unsharpness if the focal spot changes to
        1.5 mm.

3.   Calculate the amount of unsharpness if the OID changes to 4 inches.

4.   Calculate the amount of unsharpness if the SID changes to 40
        inches.

Use the factors below to answer questions 5-8:
        focal spot = 1.2 mm
        OID = 3 inches
        SID = 40 inches

5.   Calculate the amount of unsharpness.

6.   Calculate the amount of unsharpness if the focal spot changes
        .6 mm.

7.   Calculate the amount of unsharpness if the OID changes to 6 inches.

8.   Calculate the amount of unsharpness if the SID changes to 60
        inches.

Answers

1. .06	3. .04	5..10	7. .21
2. .14	4. .11	6..05	8. .06

CHAPTER 12
RADIOGRAPHIC FILM AND DEVELOPMENT

Chapter 12 continues with the discussion of recorded detail. This chapter includes most aspects of film processing.It begins with the construction of film and film types. The basics of automatic processing are next with several tables that include the essence of processing chemistry. The systems of the processor are discussed next followed by the characteristic curve and processor quality control.

If this chapter is to be used as one instructional unit, it can be broken up into five class sessions with the test given in the sixth. Some instructors may feel that this is too much material to include in one unit and may want to break the chapter up into more units.

Some suggestions are included in the introduction to this Instructor's Guide on how to vary the presentation of this chapter. Some master plans require a separate course on film processing, and the material in this chapter can easily be incorporated into the course. Some instructors may also want to save the material on the characteristic curve and processor quality control to use in a quality assurance course.

LESSON 12-1: FILM CONSTRUCTION AND
FILM TYPES

Goal
Students will be able to describe the construction of radiographic film and also the purposes for which various film types are used.

Reading Assignment
Pages 139-143

Objectives
1. List the two components of x-ray film.
2. Describe the characteristics of the film's base.
3. Describe the characteristics of the film's emulsion.
4. Differentiate between single and double emulsion film.
5. List the layers of a single and double emulsion film in order from front to back.

6. Describe the construction and uses for these types of film: screen, non-screen, periapical, occlusal, roll, 105 mm, Franklin, cinefluorography, mammography, duplicating, subtraction, and laser.

Activities

Activity 12.A   Lab performed in the darkroom to see the difference between single and double emulsion film and exposed and unexposed film

Activity 12.B   Fill-in on film construction

Activity 12.C   Clinical assignment lab on film types

Test Questions

1.   List the layers of both single- and double-emulsion film, in order, from front to back.

2.   The base of the film is called a safety base because
  a. it has rounded edges
  b. it cannot be used in acid solutions
  c. it will not burn easily
  d. it cannot be scratched

3.   The base of modern x-ray film is composed of
  a. polyester   c. silver
  b. glass   d. cardboard

4.   The emulsion of a film consists of (List all that apply.)
  a. silver bromide   c. plastic
  b. cardboard   d. gelatin
  e. polyester   f. potassium nitrate

5.   Which one of these film types would be used during a fluoroscopy exam?
  a. mammography   c. laser
  b. 105 mm   d. periapical

6.   Which one of these films requires a leader to be taped to it for processing?

a. roll film
b. screen film

c. duplicating film
d.double-emulsion film

7.   A protective coating is applied to the film's
      a. base
      b. emulsion

      c. adhesive layer
      d. supercoating

8.   Which one of these is the approximate thickness of the film base?
      a. .0005 inches
      b. .001 inches

      c. .007 inches
      d. .20 inches

9.   The blue tint that is added to the film base absorbs how much of the light from the view box?
      a. 5%
      b. 15%

      c. 85%
      d. 95%

10.   Which one of these is the advantage of the amphoteric characteristic of the gelatin used in film construction?
      a. helps the film retain its size
      b. keeps the film from burning easily
      c. allows the film to be used in both acid and alkali solutions
      d. makes the finished image more pleasing to look at

                          Answers
2. c   5. b   8. c
3. a   6. a   9. b
4. a, d   7. b   10. c

LESSON 12-2: PROCESSING AND PROCESSING CHEMICALS

Goal
Students will be able to describe the basic processing steps and the action of the processing chemicals.

Reading Assignment
Pages 144-145

Objectives

1. Name the sections involved in automatic processing in order.
2. Explain the main purpose of each processing section.
3. List the agents that are used in the developer and the fixer.
4. Describe the purpose for each of the agents in the developer and fixer.
5. Match the chemicals used with each agent in the developer and fixer.
6. List the proper temperature for developer.
7. Explain what happens to the image if the developer temperature is too high or too low.

Activities

Activity 12.D   Fill-in on processor agents and chemicals

Test Questions

1. List in order the sections of the processor that the film goes through.

2. When will the latent image be on the film?
   a. before exposure and development
   b. after exposure and development
   c. after exposure and before development
   d. before exposure and after development

3. About how long does it take to develop a film in an automatic processor?
   a. 10 seconds
   b. 20-30 seconds
   c. 45-90 seconds
   d. 2 minutes

4. Fog on the film may mean
   a. the fixer temperature was too low
   b. the dryer temperature was too high
   c. the wash temperature was too low
   d. the developer temperature was too high

5. The exposed silver bromide crystals are reduced to metallic silver in the
   a. developer
   b. fixer
   c. wash
   d. dryer

6.   The unexposed and undeveloped silver bromide crystals are removed
         in the
         a. developer   c. wash
         b. fixer   d. dryer

7.   If the developer temperature is too low the film will be
         a. light
         b. dark

Matching

8. fixing agent   a. reduces the exposed silver
                                      bromide to metallic silver

9. phenidone   b. contains potassium
                                      bromide

10. sodium sulfite   c. used as a hardener

11. accelerator   d. swells the emulsion
12. glutaraldehyde   e. preserves the life of the
                                      processing chemicals

13. hydroquinone   f. stops the action of the
                                      developer

14. ammonium thiosulfate   g. also called hypo

15. developing agent   h. removes the unexposed
                                      and undeveloped silver
                                      bromide crystals

16. fixer activator   i. chemical used as a
                                      developing agent

17. restrainer   j. develops the gray areas

Answers

2. c   6. b   10. e   14. g

73

3. c	7. a	11. d	5. a
4. d	8. h	12. c	16. f
5. a	9. j	13. l	17. b

LESSON 12-3 SYSTEMS OF THE PROCESSOR

Goal

Students will understand the functions of the roller transport and replenishment systems of the processor.

Reading Assignment

Pages 145-147

Objectives

1. List the components of the roller transport system.
2. Explain the advantage of offsetting the rollers.
3. Describe the location and function of the turnarounds and crossovers.
4. Explain the function of the guide shoes.
5. Explain how to clear a processor jam.
6. Describe how contamination of processor chemical occurs.
7. Explain the aftermath of chemical contamination.
8. Describe the special function of the entrance rollers.
9. List the processing chemicals that get replenished.
10. Explain the purpose of replenishment.

Activities

Activity 12.E   Lab performed in the darkroom with processing chemicals; allows the students to see a film being developed; requires some advance preparation

Test Questions

1.   Which one of these turns the film around at the bottom of the processor tanks?
  a. turnarounds   c. crossovers
  b. offset rollers   d. agitators

2.   Which one of these squeezes off excess chemicals before the film travels to the next section of the processor?
  a. turnarounds   c. crossovers

b. offset rollers   d. entrance rollers

3.   Which one of these turns off the safelight as the film is being
      developed?
      a. guide shoes   c. crossovers
      b. offset rollers   d. entrance rollers

4.   Which one of these controls the film feeding rate?
      a. crossovers   c. guide shoes
      b. entrance rollers   d. turnarounds

5.   Which one of these controls the replenishment rate?
      a. agitators   c. entrance rollers
      b. turnarounds   d. crossovers

6.   Which one of these helps the film turnaround at the bottom of the
      processor tanks?
      a. crossovers   c. guide shoes
      b. entrance rollers   d. offset rollers

7.   Contamination of the processor chemicals occurs when
      a. fixer is splashed into developer
      b. developer is splashed into fixer

8.   Contaminated developer chemicals
      a. must be decontaminated before using them again
      b. must be discarded
      c. are not a big problem
      d. must be replenished

9.   Which of these gets replenished?
      a. developer only
      b. fixer only
      c. both the developer and fixer

                              Answers
1. a   4. b   7. a
2. c   5. c   8. b

3. d   6. c   9. c

LESSON 12-4: THE CHARACTERISTIC CURVE

Goal
Students will be able to determine a film's speed, contrast, and exposure latitude from a characteristic curve.

Reading Assignment
Pages 147-153

Objectives
1. Explain what information can be derived from a characteristic curve.
2. State some other names for the characteristic curve.
3. Describe the three ways in which a characteristic curve can be produced.
4. Locate these parts on a graph of the characteristic curve: toe, threshold, shoulder, D-max, straight-line portion, and average gradient.
5. Explain why the toe area never drops to zero.
6. State the approximate range of image densities that will be measured by a densitometer.
7. Define the term **film speed** and explain how it is demonstrated on a characteristic curve.
8. Describe how film speed affects recorded detail.
9. Define the term **film contrast** and explain how it is demonstrated on a characteristic curve.
10. Define the term **exposure latitude** and explain how it is demonstrated on a characteristic curve.

Activities
Activity 12.F   This activity can be used with Lesson 12-4 even though it is listed in the book to follow the next lesson. The activity allows students to plot a characteristic curve.

Test Questions
For questions 1-4, you will draw a total of three characteristic curves on the same graph.

76

1. Draw a characteristic curve and label these parts: toe, threshold, shoulder, D-max, straight-line portion, and average gradient. Label the curve you drew curve "A."

2. Draw another curve labeled curve "B." This should demonstrate a film with more speed than curve "A."

3. Draw another curve labeled curve "C." This should demonstrate a film with less contrast than curve "A."

4. On curve "C," indicate where the exposure latitude is determined.

5. Base-plus-fog is measured on which part of the characteristic curve?
   a. toe   c. D-max
   b. threshold   d. straight-line portion

6. The average gradient is located on which part of the characteristic curve?
   a. toe   c. shoulder
   b. threshold   d. straight-line portion

7. Which of these are other names for the average gradient? List all that apply.
   a. slope   c. gamma
   b. base-plus-fog   d. H & D

8. The part of the characteristic curve which demonstrates when the film begins to respond to the exposure is the
   a. toe   c. shoulder
   b. threshold   d. D-max

9. If film "A" has more speed than film "B," which one of these statements is true?
   a. The slope of film "A" will be flatter than the slope of film "B."
   b. The toe of film "B" will be lower than the toe of film "A."
   c. The curve of film "A" will lie closer to the density axis than the curve of film "B."

d. The shoulder of film "A" will be lower than the shoulder of film "B."

10. If film "A" has a higher contrast than film "B," which one of these statements is true?
a. The slope of film "B" will be flatter than the slope of film "A."
b. The curve of film "A" will lie closer to the log relative exposure axis than the curve of film "B."
c. The shoulder of film "A" will be lower than the shoulder of film "B."
d. The threshold of film "B" will be lower than the toe of film "A."

11. If film "A" has a higher contrast than film "B" which one of these statements is true?
a. Film "A" will have more exposure latitude than film "B."
b. Film "B" will have more exposure latitude than film "A."

12. The highest density that a film can achieve is demonstrated by which one of these characteristic curve parts?
a. toe   c. straight-line portion
b. threshold   d. D-max

13. Recorded detail will increase with a
a. slow film speed
b. high film speed

Answers

5. a	7. a, c	9. c	11. b	13. a
6. d	8. b	10. a	12. d	

LESSON 12-5: PROCESSOR QUALITY CONTROL

Goal
Students will be able to perform quality control on a processor.

Reading Assignment
Pages 153-154

Objectives

1. Explain how speed is measured for quality control.
2. Explain how contrast is measured for quality control.
3. Explain how base-plus-fog is measured for quality control.
4. Measure speed, contrast, and base-plus-fog and plot these values on a quality control chart.
5. Analyze a quality control chart for variations in speed, contrast, and base-plus-fog.
6. List some common reasons for variations in speed, contrast and base-plus-fog.

Activities

No activities are listed in the book for this lesson, but it would be a good opportunity to show students how a clinical facility's quality control is recorded.

Activity 12.G   Chapter review

Test Questions

1. List the two pieces of equipment used to measure the values for a quality control chart.

2. List the three values that are measured for quality control.

3. Contrast is determined by
   a. subtracting a medium density step from a high density step
   b. subtracting a high density step from a medium density step
   c. adding the values of two medium density steps
   d. adding the values of a medium density step and a high density step

4. Base-plus-fog is measured
   a. on a high density step
   b. on a low density step
   c. on a medium density step
   d. on any blank area of the film

Use the following to answer questions 5-8.

A - developer temperature too high
B - developer temperature too low
C - contamination of chemicals
D - safelight fog
E - underreplenishment

List all the letters from the list above that may cause the problems listed.

5.   The film is too dark.

6.   The film is too light.

7.   Contrast is too low.

8.   Base-plus-fog is too high.

Answers

1. densitometer and sensitometer
2. speed, contrast, base-plus-fog
3. a
4. d
5. a, c, d
6. b, e
7. a, b, c, d, e
8. a, c, d

CHAPTER 13
INTENSIFYING SCREENS

Chapter 13 finishes the discussion of recorded detail. This chapter presents information on intensifying screens and imaging systems. It begins with the construction and function of the intensifying screen. The problem of light diffusion and its effect on recorded detail is next. This is followed by a discussion of the ways screen speed is increased and the effect on recorded detail. The problem of poor screen contact is next. Then the two common intensifying screen systems are discussed. The chapter then presents instruction on how to alter the mAs when screen speeds are changed. The chapter ends with a discussion of other imaging systems including direct exposure and computed radiography.

The material in this chapter can be presented in four class sessions with the test given in the fifth session. The material is not too difficult for students to comprehend, but the math component may give some students difficulty. If the clinical facilities make extensive use of direct exposure or computed radiography, the instructor may want to spend more time on these imaging systems.

LESSON 13-1: INTENSIFYING SCREEN CONSTRUCTION AND FUNCTION

Goal
Students will be able to describe the construction of an intensifying screen and describe how it functions.

Reading Assignment
Pages 157-163

Objectives
1. List the two components of an intensifying screen.
2. Describe how light is emitted by phosphors.
3. Define the terms **fluorescence** and **phosphorescence**.
4. Describe the phenomenon of light diffusion.
5. Explain how light diffusion causes a loss of recorded detail.
6. Define the term **screen speed**.
7. Explain how variations in screen speed affect density and recorded detail.

81

8. Describe the two ways in which a screen speed is changed.

Activities
No activities are associated with this lesson.

Test Questions

1. The two parts of an intensifying screen consist of
    a. a base and emulsion
    b. plasticand cardboard
    c. a base and an active layer
    d. an emulsion and an active layer

2. The ability of a material to emit light is
    a. diffusion   c. phosphorescence
    b. luminescence   d. radiation

3. The ability of a phosphor to give off light when struck by an x-ray is called
    a. luminescence   c. fluorescence
    b. afterglow   d. light diffusion

4. Continued light emission by phosphors after the x-rays have been turned off is called
    a. light diffusion   c. luminescence
    b. phosphorescence   d. luminance

5. The spreading out of light from a phosphor in all directions is called
    a. screen lag   c. phosphorescence
    b. fluorescenced   d. light diffusion

6. The ability of an intensifying screen to respond to x-ray is called
    a. luminance   c. diffusion
    b. screen speed   d. afterglow

7. Which one of the following is the major advantage associated with a high screen speed?
    a. a reduction in recorded detail
    b. a decrease in contrast

c. a reduction of the patient's radiation dose

d. a reduction of distortion

8.   An increase in screen speed causes more

a. recorded detail   c. afterglow

b. light diffusion   d. phosphorescence

9.   An increase in screen speed will result in

a. a decrease in recorded detail

b. a decrease in density

c. poor screen contact

d. a decrease in distortion

Answers

1. c	4. b	7. c
2. b	5. d	8. b
3. c	6. b	9. a

LESSON 13-2: POOR SCREEN CONTACT; SCREEN SYSTEMS

Goal

Students will be able to describe the problem associated with poor screen contact and will be able to differentiate between the two common screen systems.

Reading Assignment

Pages 162-165

Objectives

1.   Explain what causes poor screen contact.

2.   Describe how poor screen contact affects recorded detail.

3.   Describe how to test for poor screen contact.

4.   List the color of light given off by calcium tungstate screens and by rare earth screens.

5.   List the phosphors used for rare earth screens.

6.   Define the term **conversion efficiency**.

7.   Describe what is required by spectral matching.

Activities

Activity 13.A   Lab requiring x-ray exposure that requires students to perform a screen contact test

Activity 13.B   Lab requiring x-ray exposure that lets students see the light given off by different screen systems

Test Questions

1.   The ability of a phosphor to convert x-ray energy to light is called
    a. spectral matching   c. conversion efficiency
    b. radiance   d. luminescence

2.   Poor screen contact is caused by
    a. a reduction of light diffusion
    b. moving the phosphors too close to the film
    c. too much density on the film
    d. bending or warping the cassettes

3.   Poor screen contact causes
    a. an increase in contrast
    b. a decrease in recorded detail
    c. an increase in density
    d. a decrease in distortion

4.   A test for poor screen contact is performed with a
    a. wire mesh   c. penetrometer
    b. densitometer   d. sensitometer

Questions 5-10 concern the differences between calcium tungstate and rare earth intensifying screens. Label the statement with "C" if it applies to calcium tungstate screens, and "R" if it applies to rare earth screens.
    C = calcium tungstate
    R = rare earth

5.   Gives off a blue-violet light.

6.   Was developed in the 1970s.

7.   Has the best conversion efficiency.

8.   Emits a yellow-green light.

9.   May use lanthanum as a phosphor.

10.   Must use a film that is sensitive to blue light.

Answers

1. c	4. a	7. R	10. C
2. d	5. C	8. R	
3. b	6. R	9. R	

LESSON 13-3 TECHNIQUE COMPENSATION

Goal
Students will be able to alter the mAs when changing screen speeds.

Reading Assignment
Pages 165-167

Objectives
1.   Explain what other screen speed values are made relative to.
2.   Use the "to/from" system to calculate the multiplication factor for any screen speed.
3.   Use the "to/from" system to calculate the new mAs that will maintain film density when the screen speed is changed.
4.   Use the "from/to" system to calculate the new mAs that will maintain film density when the screen speed is changed.

Activities
Activity 13.C   Math practice with technique compensation
Activity 13.D   Lab requiring x-ray exposure to analyze the effect of different screen speeds on density and recorded detail

Test Questions
Calculate the new mAs that will maintain film density when the screen

85

speed is changed.

old mAs	old screen	new screen	new mAs
1. 7	100 RSV	200 RSV	_____
2. 15	300 RSV	700 RSV	_____
3. 2.5	400 RSV	200 RSV	_____
4. 50	100 RSV	600 RSV	_____
5. 12	800 RSV	200 RSV	_____
6. 4	300 RSV	50 RSV	_____
7. 1.6	500 RSV	300 RSV	_____

Answers

1. 3.5 mAs	4. 8.5 mAs	7. 2.6 mAs
2. 6.4 mAs	5. 48 mAs	
3. 5 mAs	6. 24 mAs	

LESSON 13-4: OTHER IMAGING SYSTEMS

Goal
Students will be able to describe these imaging systems: direct exposure and computed radiography.

Reading Assignment
Pages 167-171

Objectives
1. Describe how a direct exposure system functions.
2. Describe these aspects of the direct exposure system: the exposure required, the recorded detail, and radiographic contrast.
3. Describe how a computed radiography system functions.
4. Equate the terms **density, contrast,** and **recorded detail** with the similar terms used in computed radiography.
5. Define the terms **matrix** and **pixel.**
6. Explain how an image on a CRT can be adjusted to change the density, contrast, and recorded detail.

Activities

Activity 13.E   Chapter review

Test Questions

Determine whether the statements below refer to direct exposure or computed radiography.

    D = direct exposure
    C = computed radiography

1.   This system uses a computer to help form the image.

2.   This system uses a CRT.

3.   This system uses much more radiation to form the image than an intensifying screen system.

4.   This system involves a matrix and pixels.

5.   This system produces an image with low contrast.

6.   Density is referred to as brightness in this system.

7.   The image can be adjusted after the exposure with this system.

8.   This system will achieve a very high amount of recorded detail.

9.   This system will give the patient a very high dose of radiation.

10.   Density and contrast can be changed after the exposure with this system.

Answers

1. C	4. C	7. C	10. C
2. C	5. D	8. D	
3. D	6. C	9. D	

Section Review Activities

Activity 13.F   Multiple choice

Activity 13.G   Crossword puzzle
Activity 13.H   Word search

SECTION VI
RADIOGRAPHIC TECHNIQUES

CHAPTER 14
THE RELATIONSHIP OF THE
FOUR RADIOGRAPHIC QUALITIES

Chapter 14 begins a review of the four radiographic qualities. The textbook uses plus-minus charts extensively but breaks these down to very simple concepts. Only 12 factors are dealt with, and these were chosen because they are the ones the students will deal with the most in clinical situations or on the registry exam. The chapter begins with charts dealing only with density, then contrast, then recorded detail, and then distortion. The final charts put all four radiographic qualities together.

Students usually review one radiographic quality at a time with no problem. When all four radiographic qualities are on one chart the students are challenged. It is very important for the students to become adept at this, though, because when they are evaluating a radiographic image they need to evaluate all four radiographic qualities at the same time.

The material in this chapter can be presented over four class sessions with a test given in the fifth session. The tables and activities in the text can be used in the class sessions, or the activities can be assigned as homework. The format for this guide is changed for this chapter. The individual lesson plans will list the tables and activities to use in each class session and as homework assignments. Several plus-minus charts are included at the end of the instructor's chapter and these can be used for the final test for this chapter.

LESSON 14-1: DENSITY

Go over Tables 14-1 and 14-2 in class.
Assign Activities 14.1, 14.2 and 14.3 as homework.

LESSON 14-2: CONTRAST
Go over Table 14-3 and 14-4 in class.
Assign Activities 14.4, 14.5, and 14.6 as homework.

LESSON 14-3: RECORDED DETAI L AND DISTORTION
Recorded Detail
Go over Tables 14-5 and 14-6 in class.

Assign Activities 14.7, 14.8, and 14.9 as homework.

Distortion

Go over Tables 14-7 and 14-8 in class.
Assign Activities 14.10, and 14.11 as homework.

LESSON 14-4: RELATIONSHIPS OF ALL RADIOGRAPHIC QUALITIES

Go over Tables 14-9 and 14-10 in class.
Assign Activities 14.12, 14.13, 14.14, and 14.15 as homework.
The test should be just like Activities 14.12 through 14.15. The charts on pages 91-94 can be used for the test for this chapter.

Question 1

A good radiograph was produced using the factors listed. Each change is made independently. Indicate the effect on all of the radiographic qualities after each change.

+ for increase   - for decrease   0 for no change

Good radiograph:

800 mA	70 kVp	.2-mm focal spot	3.0-mm filtration
.02 sec	58" SID	5:1 grid ratio	400-speed screen
16 mAs	4" OID	14X17 collimation field size	94° dev. temp

FACTORS	DENSITY	CONTRAST	RECORDED DETAIL	DISTORTION
300 mA				
.04 sec				
5 mAs				
80 kVp				
40" SID				
8" OID				
.3-mm focal spot size				
12:1 grid ratio				
8x10 field size				
2.5-mm filtration				
50-speed screen				
90° dev. temp				

Question 2

A good radiograph was produced using the factors listed. Each change is made independently. Indicate the effect on all of the radiographic qualities after each change.

+ for increase   - for decrease   0 for no change

Good radiograph:

400 mA	80 kVp	.6-mm focal spot	2.5-mm filtration
1/40 sec	50" SID	8:1 grid ratio	300-speed screen
40 mAs	12" OID	8x10 collimation field size	95° dev. temp

FACTORS	DENSITY	CONTRAST	RECORDED DETAIL	DISTORTION
500 mA				
1/20 sec				
50 mAs				
70 kVp				
60" SID				
6" OID				
1.2-mm focal spot size				
5:1 grid ratio				
14x17 field size				
3.0-mm filtration				
200-speed screen				
98° dev. temp				

Question 3

A good radiograph was produced using the factors listed. Each change is made independently. Indicate the effect on all of the radiographic qualities after each change.

+ for increase   - for decrease   0 for no change

Good radiograph:

300 mA	80 kVp	1.2-mm focal spot	2.0-mm filtration
.015 sec	48" SID	6:1 grid ratio	50-speed screen
4.5 mAs	8" OID	10X12 collimation field size	94° dev. temp

FACTORS	DENSITY	CONTRAST	RECORDED DETAIL	DISTORTION
100 mA				
.04 sec				
6 mAs				
60 kVp				
68" SID				
2" OID				
2.0-mm focal spot size				
16:1 grid ratio				
8x10 field size				
1.2-mm filtration				
200-speed screen				
89° dev. temp				

93

Question 4

A good radiograph was produced using the factors listed. Each change is made independently. Indicate the effect on all of the radiographic qualities after each change.

+ for increase   - for decrease   O for no change

Good radiograph:

100 mA	90 kVp	1.2-mm focal spot	2.5-mm filtration
10 msec	72" SID	8:1 grid ratio	100-speed screen
1 mAs	2" OID	8X10 collimation field size	92° dev. temp

FACTORS	DENSITY	CONTRAST	RECORDED DETAIL	DISTORTION
300 mA				
25 msec				
4.7 mAs				
60 kVp				
40" SID				
9" OID				
.6-mm focal spot size				
12:1 grid ratio				
10x12 field size				
2.0-mm filtration				
500-speed screen				
98° dev. temp				

ANSWER: Question 1

A good radiograph was produced using the factors listed. Each change is made independently. Indicate the effect on all of the radiographic qualities after each change.

+ for increase   - for decrease   0 for no change

Good radiograph:

800 mA	70 kVp	1.2-mm focal spot	3.0-mm filtration
0.2 sec	58" SID	5:1 grid ratio	400-speed screen
16 mAs	4" OID	14X17 collimation field size	94° dev. temp

FACTORS	DENSITY	CONTRAST	RECORDED DETAIL	DISTORTION
300 mA	-	0	0	0
.04 sec	+	0	0	0
5 mAs	-	0	0	0
80 kVp	+	-	0	0
40" SID	+	0	-	+
8" OID	-	+	-	+
.3-mm focal spot size	0	0	+	0
12:1 grid ratio	-	+	0	0
8x10 field size	-	+	0	0
2.5-mm filtration	+	+	0	0
50-speed screen	_	0	+	0
90° dev. temp	_	_	0	0

ANSWER: Question 2

A good radiograph was produced using the factors listed. Each change is made independently. Indicate the effect on all of the radiographic qualities after each change.

+ for increase   - for decrease   0 for no change

Good radiograph:

400 mA	80 kVp	.6-mm focal spot	2.5-mm filtration
1/40 sec	50" SID	8:1 grid ratio	300-speed screen
40 mAs	12" OID	8X10 collimation field size	95° dev. temp

FACTORS	DENSITY	CONTRAST	RECORDED DETAIL	DISTORTION
500 mA	+	0	0	0
1/20 sec	+	0	0	0
50 mAs	+	0	0	0
70 kVp	-	+	0	0
60" SID	-	0	+	-
6" OID	+	-	+	-
1.2-mm focal spot	0	0	-	0
5:1 grid ratio	+	-	0	0
14X17 collimation field size	+	-	0	0
3.0-mm filtration	-	-	0	0
200 speed screen	-	0	+	0
98° dev. temp	+	-	0	0

96

ANSWER: Question 3

A good radiograph was produced using the factors listed. Each change is made independently. Indicate the effect on all of the radiographic qualities after each change.

+ for increase   - for decrease   O for no change

Good radiograph:

300 mA	80 kVp	1.2-mm focal spot	2.0-mm filtration
.015 sec	48" SID	6:1 grid ratio	50-speed screen
4.5 mAs	8" OID	10X12 collimation field size	94° dev. temp

FACTORS	DENSITY	CONTRAST	RECORDED DETAIL	DISTORTION
100 mA	-	O	O	O
.04 sec	+	O	O	O
6 mAs	+	O	O	O
60 kVp	-	+	O	O
68" SID	-	O	+	-
2" OID	+	-	+	-
2.0-mm focal spot	O	O	-	O
16:1 grid ratio	-	+	O	O
8 X 10 collimation field size	-	+	O	O
1.2-mm filtration	+	+	O	O
200-speed screen	+	O	-	O
89° dev. temp	-	-	O	O

ANSWER: Question 4

A good radiograph was produced using the factors listed. Each change is made independently. Indicate the effect on all of the radiographic qualities after each change.

+ for increase   - for decrease   0 for no change

Good radiograph:

100 mA	90 kVp	1.2-mm focal spot	2.5-mm filtration
10 msec	72" SID	8:1 grid ratio	100-speed screen
1 mAs	2" OID	8X10 collimation field size	92° dev. temp

FACTORS	DENSITY	CONTRAST	RECORDED DETAIL	DISTORTION
300 mA	+	0	0	0
25 msec	+	0	0	0
4.7 mAs	+	0	0	0
60 kVp	-	+	0	0
40" SID	+	0	-	+
9" OID	-	+	-	+
.6-mm focal spot	0	0	+	0
12:1 grid ratio	-	+	0	0
10X12 collimation field size	+	-	0	0
2.0-mm filtration	+	+	0	0
500- speed screen	+	0	-	0
98° dev. temp	+	-	0	0

CHAPTER 15
EXPOSURE COMPENSATION

Chapter 15 reviews all the math that was used in previous chapters. The following calculations are reviewed: mAs, mA, time, reciprocity, density maintenance, 15% rule, grid ratio,collimation field size, and intensifying screen speed.

The chapter can be divided into two class sessions with the test given in the third session. Students should not have too much trouble with this material if they have absorbed the math in the previous chapters.

LESSON 15-1: MATH REVIEW
During the first class session, the instructor should review all the math calculations and assign Activities 15.A, 15.B, and 15.C for homework.

LESSON 15-2: MATH REVIEW
In the second class session, the homework assignments can be corrected and any troubles ironed out. This guide includes a test that is similar to the activities that can be used for the chapter test.

Test Questions
Calculate the following:
mAs
1.   600 mA and .04 sec = _____

2.   200 mA and 2/15 sec = _____

3.   What mAs is achieved with an mA or 300 and a time of .025 sec?

     _____

mA
4.   40 mAs and .20 sec = _____

5.   20 mAs and 1/40 sec = _____

6.   If a mAs of 10 is desired at a time station of .025 sec, what mA station would be necessary? _____

Time
7.   12 mAs and 300 mA = _____

8.   9 mAs and 600 mA = _____

9.   If 400 mA is used to produce 10 mAs, what time station must be
        used? _____

Use these mA and time station for problems 10-13:

mA	Time	
25 small focal spot	.01	.30
50	.02	.40
100	.025	.50
200	.03	.70
300 large focal spot	.05	1.0
400	.10	2.0
500	.15	3.0
600	.20	4.0
		5.0

Reciprocity

10.   List 3 sets of mA and time that would produce 15 mAs.
        mA _____ time
        mA _____ time
        mA _____ time

11.   The original exposure factors are 500 mA and .25 sec. Change this
        to a breathing technique.
        mA _____ time _____

12.   The original exposure factors are 100 mA and .3 sec. Change this
        to a better technique to control motion.
        MA _____ time _____

13.   The original exposure factors are 400 mA and .05 sec. Change
        this to a   technique that would produce better recorded detail.
        MA _____ time _____

The Density Maintenance Formula

	new mAs	old mAs	new distance	old distance
14.	____	15	72	40
15.	____	4	66	44

100

16. The SID is changed from 72 inches to 60 inches. The original mAs was14. What new mAs is required to maintain film density at the new SID?

The 15% Rule

	new kVp	new mAs	old mAs	old kVp
17.	_____	12	24	75
18.	70	_____	6.2	80

19. The original exposure factors are 3 mAs at 90 kVp. Using the 15% rule, change this to a technique that would produce higher contrast.

20. The original exposure factors are 300 mA, .5 sec., at 70 kVp. Using the 15% rule, change this to a technique that would control motion better.

Grid Ratio

	new mAs	old mAs	old grid ratio	new grid ratio
21.	_____	8	8:1	16:1
22.	_____	7.5	12:1	6:1
23.	_____	4.2	16:1	8:1

24. The original mAs of 9 was used with a 6:1 grid ratio. If the grid ratio is changed to a 12:1, what new mAs would be required to maintain the original radiographic density?

Collimation Field Size

	new mAs	old mAs	old field size	new field size
25.	_____	12	10 X 12	14 X 17
26.	_____	7	8 X 10	10 X 12

27. A KUB was taken on a 14 X 17 using 4.6 mAs at 70 kVp. The radiologist wants a "coned down" view of the right upper quadrant on an 8 X 10. What new mAs would be required?

Intensifying Screen Speed

	multiplication factor	screen speed
28.	_____	500
29.	_____	100

new mAs	old mAs	old screen speed	new screen speed
30.____	10	200	400
31.____	3	600	200

32. The ordinary technique for a lateral cervical spine is 500 mA, .01 sec., and 70 kVp on a 100-speed intensifying screen. Motion is likely to be a problem on this patient, so a 400-speed intensifying screen is used. What new mAs is required?

33. An AP shoulder is performed at 3 mAs and 75 kVp using a 400-speed screen. The radiologist suspects a bony lesion at the humeral shaft and needs a film with good recorded detail. It is decided to change to a screen with a speed of 100. What new mAs is required?

Answers

1. 24 mAs
2. 27 mAs
3. 7.5 mAs

4. 200 mA
5. 800 mA
6. 400 mA
7. .04 sec.
8. .015 sec.
9. .025 sec.
10. any mA and time to equal 15 mAs
11. 25 mA, 5 sec.
12. 600 mA, .05 sec.
13. 200 mA, .10 sec.
14. 48.6 mAs
15. 9 mAs
16. 9.7 mAs
17. 85 kVp
18. 12.4 mAs
19. 6 mAs, 80 kVp
20. 300 mA, .25 sec., 80 kVp
21. 12 mAs
22. 4.5 mAs
23. 2.8 mAs
24. 15 mAs
25. 9.6 mAs
26. 6.25 mAs
27. 6.4 mAs
28. .2
29. 1
30. 5 mAs
31. 8.8 mAs
32. 1.25 mAs
33. 12 mAs

CHAPTER 16
TECHNIQUE
CONVERSION AND COMPARISON

Chapter 16 expands on the math review presented in Chapter 15. Two types of problems are included in this chapter. One type is technique conversions that involve several changes simultaneously. This is a type of problem that students are often presented with in clinical situations especially when changing from a routine procedure to a portable exam. In the second type of problem the student is given four sets of exposure conditions and must calculate which set will produce the greatest or least density. Several of these problems are usually included in the ARRT exam. The chapter gives students detailed information on how to calculate both of these problems.

This guide lists the activities in the book that should be used during class sessions and as homework assignments. The material in this chapter can be covered in three class sessions with the fourth session for the test. The guide gives the instructor a test that can be used for the chapter test.

LESSON 16-1: CONVERSION PROBLEMS
The instructor should show the students how to calculate conversion problems. Activities 16.A and 16.B can then be assigned as homework.

LESSON 16-2: COMPARISON PROBLEMS
The instructor should show . the students how to calculate comparison problems. Then activities 16.C and 16.D can be assigned as homework.

LESSON 16-3: REVIEW
It is suggested that this class session be used to correct homework problems and to see if students are having any difficulty with either type of problem.

Test Questions

	A		B	
1.	100	mA	400	mA
	1/4	sec	_____	sec
	8:1	grid	12:1	grid
	50"	SID	40"	SID

2. | 200 | mA | | | _____ | mA |
    |-----|-----|---|---|-------|-----|
    | .15 | sec | | | .10 | sec |
    | 76 | kVp | | | 86 | kVp |
    | 300 | RSV | | | 600 | RSV |

3. | 200 | mA | | 600 | mA |
    |-----|-----|---|-----|-----|
    | .05 | sec | | _____ | sec |
    | 68" | SID | | 42" | SID |
    | 200 | RSV | | 500 | RSV |

4. | 300 | mA | | _____ | mA |
    |-----|-----|---|-------|-----|
    | 1/30 | sec | | 1/20 | sec |
    | 68 | kVp | | 78 | kVp |
    | 56" | SID | | 48" | SID |
    | 16:1 | grid | | 8:1 | grid |

5. | 15 | mAs | | _____ | mAs |
    |-----|-----|---|-------|-----|
    | 40" | SID | | 48" | SID |
    | 80 | kVp | | 90 | kVp |
    | 12:1 | grid | | 5:1 | grid |
    | 8X10 | collimation | | 14X17 | collimation |

6. | 100 | mA | | 100 | mA |
    |-----|-----|---|-----|-----|
    | 1/2 | sec | | _____ | sec |
    | 70 | kVp | | 80 | kVp |
    | 12:1 | grid | | 6:1 | grid |
    | 200 | RSV | | 400 | RSV |

7. | 60 | mAs | | _____ | mAs |
    |-----|-----|---|-------|-----|
    | 82 | kVp | | 72 | kVp |
    | 14X17 | collimation | | 10X12 | collimation |
    | 70" | SID | | 42" | SID |

8. | 45 | mAs | | _____ | mAs |
    |-----|-----|---|-------|-----|
    | 6:1 | grid | | 12:1 | grid |
    | 100 | RSV | | 600 | RSV |
    | 44" | SID | | 68" | SID |

9.
100 mA		400 mA
.3 sec		_____ sec
48" SID		72" SID
60 kVp		70 kVp
16:1 grid		6:1 grid

10.   Which one of these exposures would produce the *greatest* density?

A	B	C	D
400 mA	400 mA	100mA	200 mA
.2 sec	.1 sec	.4 sec	.5 sec
90 kVp	80 kVp	90 kVp	80 kVp
16:1 grid	5:1 grid	16:1 grid	8:1 grid
40" SID	44" SID	36" SID	72" SID

11.   Which one of these exposures would produce the *greatest* density?

A	B	C	D
200 mA	200 mA	400 mA	100 mA
1/2 sec	1/4 sec	1/15 sec	1/10 sec
48" SID	36" SID	42" SID	66" SID
80 kVp	90 kVp	70 kVp	80 kVp
16:1grid	12:1 grid	16:1 grid	6:1 grid
100 RSV	300 RSV	500 RSV	100 RSV

12.   Which one of these exposures would produce the *least* density?

A	B	C	D
100 mA	300 mA	400 mA	500 mA
30 msec	50 msec	25 msec	15 msec
70 kVp	80 kVp	90 kVp	80 kVp
36" SID	58" SID	44" SID	65" SID
100 RSV	800 RSV	200 RSV	300 RSV

13.　Which one of these exposures would produce the *least* density?

A	B	C	D
100 mA	300 mA	50 mA	200 mA
1/2 sec	1/5 sec	1 sec	1/4 sec
70 kVp	80 kVp	70 kVp	80 kVp
40" SID	58"SID	44" SID	66" SID

14.　Which one of these exposures would produce the *greatest* density?

A	B	C	D
1000 mA	100 mA	800 mA	400 mA
.2 sec	.7 sec	.15 sec.	25 sec
90 kVp	70 kVp	80 kVp	80 kVp
16:1 grid	12:1grid	6:1 grid	8:1 grid
10X12 coll.	8X10 coll.	14X17 coll.	14X17 coll.

Answers

1. .05 sec	5. 3 mAs	9. .04 sec	13. D
2. 77 mA	6. .075 sec	10. A	14. A
3. .0025 sec	7. 54 mAs	11. A	
4. 49 mA	8. 31 mAs	12. A	

CHAPTER 17
RADIOGRAPHIC TECHNIQUE CHARTS

Chapter 17 presents the subject of technique charts. It begins by analyzing the two most common types of charts: the fixed kVp and the variable kVp chart. The reasons why the fixed kVp chart is generally preferred over the variable kVp chart are discussed. Radiographers must know when to alter the technique suggested by the fixed kVp chart, and these instances are analyzed.

The material in this chapter is not too difficult for students. The chapter can be presented in two class sessions with a test given in the third session.

LESSON 17-1: TYPE OF TECHNIQUE CHARTS

Goal
Students will be able to describe the two types of technique charts and use a fixed kVp chart.

Reading Assignment
Pages 205-211

Objectives
1. Describe the two most common technique charts.
2. Explain what is varied and what is fixed on each chart.
3. Measure a body part with a caliper.
4. State which chart uses optimum kVp.
5. Explain why a technique from a fixed kVp chart will always penetrate the body part, produce sufficient radiographic contrast, and produce an acceptable level of scattered radiation.
6. Describe how a fixed kVp chart yields these advantages: lower radiation dose to the patient, higher exposure latitude, and better ability to control motion.
7. Explain how to produce a technique chart.

Activities
No activities are associated with this lesson.

Test Questions
For questions 1-15, indicate whether the statement refers to a fixed kVp

chart, a variable kVp chart, both a fixed and variable kVp chart, or neither a fixed or variable kVp chart.

> F = fixed kVp chart
> V = variable kVp chart
> B = both fixed and variable kVp charts
> N = neither a fixed or variable kVp chart

1. The kVp might not penetrate the part.

2. Increases size distortion.

3. Uses optimum kVp.

4. Tends to use higher kVp values.

5. kVp should be varied according to the patient's body size.

6. Usually produces a lower patient dose.

7. Density will always be too low.

8. The user of the chart should measure the patient's body part.

9. Can only be used with calcium tungstate intensifying screens.

10. Only varies the mAs for body parts of different size.

11. Tends to produce an image with higher contrast.

12. Reduces the need for good quality control of the processor.

13. Produces an acceptable amount of scattered radiation.

14. The radiographer must collimate to the size of the film.

15. This is the type of chart used in your clinical assignment.

Answers

1. V	6. F	11. V
2. N	7. N	12. N

3. F   8. B   13. F
4. F   9. N   14. B
5. V   10. F   15. the chart used clinically

LESSON 17-2: ALTERING TECHNIQUES

Goal
Students will be able to vary the technique suggested by the technique chart when necessary.

Reading Assignment
Pages 211-213

Objectives
1. State how often a correctly formulated technique chart will be accurate.
2. Explain how to alter the technique when the patient's physical condition is very different from average.
3. List the pathologies that require the technique to be increased from what is suggested by the chart.
4. List the pathologies that require the technique to be decreased from what is suggested by the chart.

Activities
Activity 17.A   Chapter review

Test Questions
For questions 1-15, indicate whether the technique on the chart should be used or the technique should be increased, decreased from what is suggested by the chart.

C = use the technique on the chart
I = increase the technique from the chart
D = decrease the technique from the chart

1.   The patient is in the early stages of emphysema.

2.   The patient is of average physique.

3.   The patient has a possible fracture of the ankle with no evidence of edema.

4.   The patient has ascites.

5.   The patient has multiple myeloma.

6.   The patient has a bowel obstruction with a large amount of gas.

7.   The patient has an increased muscular development.

8.   The patient measures more than the highest category listed on the chart.

9.   The patient has Paget's disease.

10.   The patient has metastasis to the bone.

11.   The patient has pneumonia.

12.   The patient has pulmonary edema.

13.   The patient has pleural effusion.

14.   The patient has osteoporosis.

15.   The patient has congestive heart failure.

Answers

1. D	6. D	11. I
2. C	7. I	12. I
3. C	8. I	13. I
4. I	9. I	14. D
5. D	10. D	15. I

CHAPTER 18
AUTOMATIC EXPOSURE CONTROL

Chapter 18 presents the subject of automatic exposure control or phototiming. It begins by describing how a photocell functions. Then the chapter describes how these aspects of automatic exposure control should be used: the backup time, kVp, mA, photocell arrangement, the body part position, and automatic exposure control density settings. Minimum reaction time is also discussed.

The material in this chapter may be difficult for students who have not used automatic exposure control clinically. The chapter can be presented in two class sessions with a test given in the third session.

LESSON 18-1: AUTOMATIC EXPOSURE CONTROL TECHNIQUE

Goal

Students will be able to use these three aspects of automatic exposure control: backup time, kVp, and mA.

Reading Assignment

Pages 215-218

Objectives

1. Define automatic exposure control.
2. Explain how a photocell functions.
3. Describe how high the backup time should be set.
4. Explain why optimum kVp should be used with automatic exposure control.
5. Explain what happens if the optimum kVp is not used for automatic exposure control.
6. Explain how the mA should be selected when using automatic exposure control.

Activities

No activities are associated with this lesson.

Test Questions

1. If the ordinary exposure time for a KUB is .15 sec, how high must the backup time be set?
    a. above .15 sec
    b. below .15 sec

2.   Which one of these determines the length of time for an exposure made with automatic exposure control?
a. the type of photocell used
b. the amount of exit radiation hitting the photocell
c. the amount of primary radiation used
d. all of the above

For questions 3-6 this is the automatic exposure control technique used:
400 mA
80 kVp
.5 sec backup time

Indicate how the automatic exposure control will respond or how the image will be affected with the following changes:

3.   The kVp is increased to 90
a. the mA will be increased
b. the density will increase
c. the contrast will decrease
d. recorded detail will increase

4.   The mA is decreased to 300
a. the time will be increased
b. kVp will be decreased
c. the time will be decreased
d. kVp will be increased

5.   The backup time is increased to 1.0 sec
a. kVp will be decreased
b. mA will be increased
c. contrast will increase
d. this change will have no effect

6.   The mA is increased to 600
a. kVp will be decreased
b. there will be more distortion on the image
. c. the exposure time will be decreased
d. recorded detail will decrease

Answers

1. a	3. c	5. d
2. b	4. a	6. c

112

LESSON 18-2: POSITIONING WITH
AUTOMATIC EXPOSURE CONTROL

Goal

Students will be able to position the body part correctly when using automatic exposure control.

Reading Assignment

Pages 218-223

Objectives

1. Explain how the 3 photocells are arranged.
2. Describe how the photocell arrangement should be selected for common radiographic procedures.
3. Explain why the photocell must be completely covered by the body part.
4. Explain why the body part to be demonstrated must be positioned over the photocell.
5. Explain how the automatic exposure control density can be adjusted to alter radiographic density.
6. Explain how the minimum reaction time of automatic exposure control can affect the length of the exposure.

Activities

Activity 18.A   Lab requiring x-ray exposure to analyze photocell arrangement

Activity 18.B   Lab requiring x-ray exposure to analyze the effect of covering the photocell with the body part

Activity 18.C   Lab requiring x-ray exposure to analyze the effect of centering of the body part over the photocell

Activity 18.D   Chapter review

Test Questions

1. Which photocell arrangement should be selected for a KUB?
   a. the 2 outside photocells
   b. the center photocell

2. Which photocell arrangement should be selected for a PA chest?
   a. the 2 outside photocells
   b. the center photocell

3. Which photocell arrangement should be selected for a lateral chest?
    a. the 2 outside photocells
    b. the center photocell

4. Which photocell arrangement should be selected for an AP shoulder?
    a. the 2 outside photocells
    b. the center photocell

5. If an AP hip is positioned so that the photocell is not completely
    covered by the body part, what is likely to happen to the image?
    a. it will be too light
    b. it will be too dark

6. If a lateral stomach with barium is positioned so that the barium is
    not centered over the photocell, what is likely to happen to the
    image?
    a. it will be too light
    b. it will be too dark

7. The automatic exposure control density should be set one step lower
    for which one of these patients?
    a. a patient of average physique
    b. a patient of high muscular physique
    c. an emaciated patient

8. Adjusting kVp with automatic exposure control changes which one
    of these radiographic qualities?
    a. density   c. recorded detail
    b. contrast   d. distortion

9. If the backup time is not set above the minimum reaction time,
    which result will occur?
    a. the image will be too light
    b. the image will be too dark

Answers

1. a	4. b	7. c
2. a	5. a	8. b
3. b	6. a	9. a

APPENDIX A
BASIC MATH REVIEW

MATH TEST

Fractions

1. $500 \times \dfrac{2}{5} =$

2. $25 \times \dfrac{5}{6} =$

3. $100 \times \dfrac{7}{8} =$

4. $1200 \times \dfrac{2}{3} =$

5. $200 \div \dfrac{2}{3} =$

6. $400 \div \dfrac{1}{4} =$

7. $50 \div \dfrac{3}{5} =$

8. $1000 \div \dfrac{1}{2} =$

9. $\dfrac{1}{2} + \dfrac{2}{3} + \dfrac{4}{6} =$

10. $\dfrac{2}{3} + \dfrac{6}{8} + \dfrac{12}{16} =$

11. $\dfrac{3}{4} + \dfrac{6}{12} + \dfrac{8}{15} =$

12. $\dfrac{1}{5} + \dfrac{7}{8} + \dfrac{5}{4} =$

13. $\dfrac{3}{4} - \dfrac{6}{12} =$

14. $\dfrac{5}{6} - \dfrac{8}{14} =$

15. $\dfrac{7}{8} - \dfrac{3}{5} =$

16. $\dfrac{9}{11} - \dfrac{4}{7} =$

17. $\dfrac{3}{4} \times \dfrac{2}{3} =$

18. $\dfrac{10}{12} \times \dfrac{6}{8} =$

19. $\dfrac{5}{4} \times \dfrac{3}{6} =$

20. $\dfrac{6}{8} \times \dfrac{7}{9} =$

21. $\dfrac{3}{4} \div \dfrac{5}{6} =$ 22. $\dfrac{10}{14} \div \dfrac{9}{7} =$

23. $\dfrac{2}{3} \div \dfrac{4}{5} =$ 24. $\dfrac{8}{3} \div \dfrac{7}{9} =$

Decimals

25. 4.535
      .734
     3.800
   +   .007

26. 5.790
     1.256
      .530
   + .092

27.   Add these numbers: 1.276, .35, .008, 1.56

28.   Add these numbers: 5.6, .40, 1.259, .05

29.   387.5
       - 45.9

30. .006
    - .003

31. Subtract these numbers: 6.463 minus 2.673

32. Subtract 4.594 from 6.395

33.   .458
       X .500

34. .238
    X .482

35.   Multiply 4.698 by 2.964

36.   Multiply .75 by 7.345

37. $.55\overline{)1.75}$ 38. $.6\overline{)1.45}$

39.   Divide .167 by .20

40.   Divide 4.92 by .3

41.   Convert .25 to a fraction

116

42.   Convert .004 to a fraction

43.   Convert .87 to a fraction

44.   Convert .2 to a fraction

45.   Convert this fraction to a decimal $\dfrac{1}{8}$

46.   Convert this fraction to a decimal $\dfrac{90}{240}$

47.   Convert this fraction to a decimal $\dfrac{234}{569}$

48.   Convert this fraction to a decimal $\dfrac{1500}{300}$

Percentage

49.   Convert this percentage to a decimal   10%

50.   Convert this percentage to a decimal   250%

51.   Convert this percentage to a decimal   3%

52.   Convert this percentage to a decimal   1480%

53.   Convert this decimal to a percentage   .45

54.   Convert this decimal to a percentage   .07

55.   Convert this decimal to a percentage   3.58

56.   Convert this decimal to a percentage   .006

57.   Convert this percentage to a fraction   25%

58.   Convert this percentage to a fraction   345%

59.   Convert this percentage to a fraction 6%

60.   Convert this percentage to a fraction .5%

61.   Convert this fraction to a percentage $\dfrac{1}{2}$

62.   Convert this fraction to a percentage $\dfrac{35}{50}$

63.   Convert this fraction to a percentage $\dfrac{456}{948}$

64.   Convert this fraction to a percentage $\dfrac{14}{16}$

65.   Increase 400 by 50%

66.   Increase 70 by 15%

67.   Decrease 120 by 24%

68.   Decrease 86 by 6%

Algebra
Solve for x
69.   x + 6 = 58

70.   x + 25 = 678
71.   x - 7 = 45

72.   x - 15 = 53

73.   x = 5(3) + 35

74.   x = 46 + 4(3)

75.   x = 6(45 + 68 - 72)

76.   x = 7(36 - 74 + 42)

77.   x = (80 ÷ 32) + 56(2 + 25) - 3

78.   x = 6(34-28) + 105 - (45 + 29)

Ratios and Proportions
Solve for x

79. $\dfrac{x}{4} = \dfrac{2}{8}$

80. $\dfrac{7}{x} = \dfrac{2}{14}$

81. $\dfrac{3}{12} = \dfrac{9}{x}$

82. $\dfrac{8}{4} = \dfrac{x}{2}$

Exponents

83. $x^2 = 64$

84. $x^2 = 625$

85. $8^3 =$

86. $10^{-1} =$

Answers

1. 200	23. 5/6	45. .125	67. 91.2
2. 20.8	24. 3.43	46. .375	68. 80.84
3. 87.5	25. 9.076	47. .41	69. 52
4. 800	26. 7.668	48. 5	70. 653
5. 300	27. 3.194	49. .1	71. 52
6. 1600	28. 7.309	50. 2.5	72. 68
7. 83.3	29. 341.6	51. .03	73. 50
8. 2000	30. .003	52. 14.80	74. 58
9. 1.83	31. 3.79	53. 45%	75. 246
10. 2.17	32. 1.801	54. 7%	76. 28
11. 1.78	33. .229	55. 358%	77. 1511.5
12. 2.325	34. .114716	56. .6%	78. 67
13. 1/4	35. 13.93	57. 1/4	79. 1
14. 11/42	36. 5.50875	58. 69/200	80. 49
15. 11/40	37. 3.18	59. 3/50	81. 36
16. 19/77	38. 2.417	60. 1/200	82. 4
17. 1/2	39. .835	61. 50%	83. 8
18. 5/8	40. 16.4	62. 70%	84. 25
19. 5/8	41. 1/4	63. 48.1%	85. 512
20. 7/12	42. 1/250	64. 87.5%	86. 1
21. 9/10	43. 87/100	65. 600	
22. 5/9	44. 1/5	66. 80.5